The Theory of Natural Systems

Genetic Immunity and the cure of cancer and AIDS

by

Maria L. Costell Gaydos

First published by AuthorHouse 07/02/04

ISBN: 1-4184-7816-4 (e-book)
ISBN: 1-4184-4130-9 (Paperback)

This book is printed on acid free paper.

TABLE OF CONTENTS

FREEDOM,
THE PILLAR OF THE UNIVERSE.

Que ley, justicia o razón	What law, justice or reason
negar a los hombres sabe	can deny men
privilegio tan suave,	so subtle privilege
exceptión tan principal,	exception so fundamental,
qu Dios le ha dado a un cristal,	that God has given to a crystal,
a un pez, a un bruto y a un ave?	a fish, a brute and a bird?

Calderón de la Barca. (La Vida es Sueño)

"Freedom of decision, the *power to decide its* own course of action or inaction is inherent to every being of the universe." This postulate will be reasoned and repetitively illustrated in this thesis. Freedom of decision shall be clearly differentiated from freedom of action. While a prisoner is not free to act as he pleases, he is always free to make his decisions. This is a capability inextricably embodied in his own being, and this thesis propounds that such is also a capability of every other creature and thing.

The notion that freedom shall not be confined to man is not new but it has not been debated to be a *universal* essence of nature. That will change our present views of physical reality. Calderón de la Barca, Spanish poet-philosopher of the seventieth century, openly attributed "freedom" to "a crystal, a fish, a brute and a bird." At that time to postulate that things and creatures have power of decision was to confront the basic beliefs of that age. Then, religion, philosophical tradition and government institutions considered man to be the lord of creation and the only creature endowed with a responsible soul, that is, *free to decide.* This exalted idea of man was a doctrine poorly enforced even in Judeo-Christianity where legal slavery was still to be practiced for several more centuries.

Today, with overwhelming information at reach, we cannot continue to sustain the notion that man, being:

- a *product* of the universe,
- *embedded* in the universe,
- *supported* by the same universe of every other creature that populates it,

has *the power to decide* on his own while the rest of the universe is deprived of such a power. Is this not an absurd, baseless and arrogant doctrine?

Experience supports the opposite. "You can bring a horse to a river but you cannot force him to drink the water." Here you have it! The horse decides by himself. In the entire universe, there is no line of demarcation indicating where or when *freedom* appears or disappears.

The *universe* is consistent with itself and this demands that freedom be fundamental and essential to all its creatures, from those created in the Big Bang to those existing in our present day. *Freedom of decision* did not appear with man. The Creation evolves and likewise *freedom of decision* in creatures and in things evolves parallel to the complexity of their systems.

Obviously *free decisions* are a matter of *qualified* degree. Free decisions of elemental particles are limited to minimum choices: the management of their systems and association with other particles. Atoms require higher levels of freedom of decision to meet complex management of protons, neutrons, electrons and selection of other atoms to form molecules. Freedom further evolves in molecules from inorganic to organic chemistry. Later, it transcends in organized systems, living systems, and man. *Freedom of decision* becomes increasingly noticeable as evolution progresses and it becomes indisputable in man. Nevertheless in simpler expression it is present in all beings, and it is needed by all systems to exist and to evolve to superior ones.

This thesis postulates that besides *freedom of decision*, things and creatures have capability to make *meaning* out of information. That is, in the inexhaustible wealth of information of the universe, they process only from **that** information which has *meaning* for their own systems and that can be processed by their own systems. While elemental particles deal with very limited energy and matter, complex systems deal with wider ranges of useful information. They are equipped with the capacity to process and to draw *meaning* from **that** information. A horse will not have use for the alphabet or the symphony of Beethoven; characters and notes are meaningless to him. There is required the intelligence of a writer or a musician to make sense or meaning of such information. Capability to draw *meaning from information* necessarily evolves with the evolvement of the organization. Thus there are a specific level of information that each organization can process and a specific level of action that they may decide to take.

The faculty to make *meaning* of information is needed by all physical reality to regulate their actions and functions, that is, to decide. Living creatures are endowed with intelligence of survival, of survival of the species, and of evolutionary impulse. Down the scale, elemental particles have the same need and for the same reasons: individual existence and evolution. Things and creatures, although they may be pressed to take a course of action dictated by the right interpretation of information, still they are free to decide otherwise or just contrary to it. The horse we bring to the river might decide not to drink water for no reason whatsoever even if he were thirsty and other horses would drink in his same circumstances. It is his choice, his *free decision.* While *meaning* is precisely bound to information, as mirrors precisely reflect images, no *decision* of any creature is *deterministically* bound to the *meaning* they draw from information. Nor their *decisions* are *bound* to any other factor or variable. Therefore *freedom of decision* can be deemed to be **the ultimate variable of the universe, the propeller of action in the Creation.** It is *supreme* in each system and totally *independent* from any other system.

We will see that the very existence of the universe would not be possible without the *freedom of decision* of all things and creatures. It will **not** be possible:

- the *unequal distribution* of matter and energy that depends upon the individual traveling of quanta of energy and matter,
- the *association of elemental matter* into atoms, molecules, and systems that depends on the selection of partners,
- *intelligent processes and functions* that preclude the interminable failures of *chance,*

- *evolution and creation* of things and creatures
  that is the mark of purpose and action, or
- *the speed* at which these miracles take place.
  In order for these happenings to take place *by
  chance* -if at all possible- would take billions
  times the age of the universe.

The universe cannot be rationalized if *freedom of
decision* is not fundamentally implanted in physical
reality. No doubt that the Creation was miraculous long
before the gift of *free will* to man.

We will see that the Laws of Nature are *not* immutable
mandates imposed upon the universe. Mandates make no
sense among creatures that draw *meaning* from information
and are *free to decide*. How, when and from where these
laws come if they are considered independent entities?
How they evolve from the laws that regulated the
universe just born in the Big Bang to those that later
appear to govern a universe twenty billion years old,
expanded beyond imagination and populated with most
intricate and diverse creatures? The so named laws of
nature are nothing else than *descriptions* of the *general*
behavior of physical reality. Such behavior is not
universally uniform because freedom of decision of all
creatures allows them not to follow the *general* behavior
of the rest who follow the logical interpretation of
information. Only *freedom of decision* and capability to
make meaning of information are <u>universal</u> fundaments of

things and creatures, **essential** to their identities and as such _intransferable_ from one being to another. (Any transferable reality be it elemental particle, atom, molecule, living being or cosmic structure is to be considered _information_ for the purposes of this theory as it will be explained later).

Both capacities, _freedom of decision_ and _to make meaning from information_, are needed. One of them will not make sense without the other. Why would nature make creatures able to make _meaning_ from information if they were unable to decide upon it? Such capacity would be useless for _indecisive_ creatures. They would be left in the hands of innumerable and mostly unsuccessful trials of _chance_ to produce new organizations. Why would nature provide creatures with _power to decide_ upon information that is _meaningless_ to them? These _decisive_ creatures would do blind and purposeless decisions and the information of the entire universe would be a waste. Evolution would be totally impossible for random processes do not qualify as evolutionary processes under any rational light. Nature does not waste resources, and such proposition will be nothing else than the waste of all the information the entire universe can provide.

Most of the matter of the cosmos is assembled in galaxies, immense clusters of celestial structures made up of compact associations of matter. The drive of matter _to associate_ manifests itself in the macro as well as in the microworld of elemental particles, atoms, and molecules. On Earth the process escalates to the creation of life and man. But there are still elemental particles in the cosmic spaces that stand *unassociated* despite the *general trend of matter to associate* in stellar formations of unimaginable-pressured matter and energy. That is the case of the light that pervades the Creation. This partial isolation of physical realities proves the existence of *individual freedom of decision.* The *unassociated* particles could have followed the *normal social tendencies of matter,* and yet, as the thirsty donkey that refused to drink water when most donkeys would, they *decided* to remain alone. And the rest of the universe could not change *their decision.* Individual freedom of decision remains the ultimate variable for all creatures of the universe. **Upon the pillar of freedom of decision the universe was and is born every fraction of a second evolving the creation of new physical realities.**

CHAPTER I. - IDENTITY AS FUNDAMENTAL ESSENCE OF PHYSICAL REALITY

PERCEPTION OF REALITY. - IDENTITY.

Reality seems to play a game with man's efforts to name, investigate and classify the countless creatures and objects of his surroundings, for no sooner than the items are individually perceived, it is realized that such items are rather *groupings* of simpler ones that are worlds on their own. In the *naming,* however, there is implicit the *notion* of *identity,* a complex construct that acknowledges the existence and uniqueness of the creature, whole and parts, functions and structure: its *real identity.* The subdivision of matter in simpler and smaller components has been going on for centuries up to the present times when probing in the microworld

1

of elemental matter seems to have reached the ultimate limits. The division of particles do not render what may be termed components or parts instead they become transformed into others, or even into each other, by addition or emission of energy. Actually, the creation of particles out of nothing, and even their annihilation, has been observed. The very specialized field of high-energy physics and subatomic particles is far from our reach although we occasionally will refer to it.

This planet, and the universe as well, is a complex labyrinth of intermingling systems into systems, and what appears to be a *unity* to the senses may be discovered to be a collection of other *unities* if submitted to magnification. To add to the confusion a slight change in observation devises will suffice to throw the observer into unexpected dimensions. We find ourselves deeper and deeper in this situation with the advances of instrumentation. When an object is illuminated by ordinary light, x-rays, or a beam of electrons the exposures yielded are practically unrelated. Nowadays we can pose for a portrait of bust, bones or cellular structures by switching on the appropriate lighting or radiation. Each of these images being one aspect of a unique reality: our *identity*.

In the middle of this perceptual confusion of reality we cling to our beliefs that creatures and things are *unities* possessing an individuality -each of them- in spite of their components or the ways they are observed. There is something beyond division or perception that imparts distinctiveness and personality to things and creatures no matter how similar they might be or to subjects as disparate as a star, an atom, a man, a family or a city, including the case when one is part of the other. *That* is their own *identity*. The rest of the creation seems to participate in this notion to judge by the *selective* interaction with their surroundings. There would be no *selectivity* in absence of *identity*.

The *identity* of each being is above its own components, set apart as a *non-transferable* entity of clear uniqueness and imposing reality. *Identity* eludes measurements, weight, dissection or analysis. It rests in the *abstract*. It is something distinct from matter or action but emerging from it. How can the nature of *identity* be described? To be *non-transferable* is a very specific attribute but not enough for description. There are other features of physical reality that are also non-transferable like sensations of pain and pleasure. How did *identity* originate? What is it made of? In what dimensions is it located? How does operate? What is the fundamental character of this *self-manifested reality* that seems to be *essential* to every being of the creation?

We will try to convey along this theory that *identity* is perceived by all creatures and physical realities throughout an immaterial process that recognizes both *self-identity* and *other's identity*.

ABOUT THE IDENTITIES OF GROUPS.

Let's reflect on what makes a group of components appear as a singular being with a clear *identity* whether it is a *natural* occurrence such as a cosmic constellation, a living creature, a crystal, or an *artificial* one devised by man as a civic organization or an instrument.

At first sight we observe that the *identity* of an aggregation of elements is an entity that differs in essence and properties from its components. The *whole* cannot be equated to its parts. Not even the mere accumulation of parts makes up a distinct unity entitled to be deemed an *individual* endowed with *identity*. The identity named *family* is endowed with specific relations among its members in addition to the people that constitute it. These people striped of their mutual relationships will not make a family. The scattered pieces of a car, however perfect they might be, will not bring you half a mile along the road, as a car should. That belongs to the identity *car*. The artist that paints a rose with skillful strokes of color creates a piece of art, an *identity*, a quality not encased in the chemical pigments. Thus, besides the components of the group there are relationships among them that gives the

4

group the structure needed to produce a novel *identity*, be it an instrument, man made organization, or natural creature.

The *group-relations* in the previous examples are *not tangible* items in part or in their totality. Although the whole system and components are concrete realities, the *relationships* between the components are links that reside in the field of emotions, intelligences, wills and creation, and these are *intangible, immaterial*. The family links are complex human relations grounded in nature or society; the design of the car is an intelligent plan imposed upon the parts; the rose picture reflects the emotional and creative faculties of the artist translated into shapes and colors.

There are fundamental differences between identities of *artificial* and *natural* associations. In the artificial ones the relations among the parts are imposed by external agents according to intelligent plans. In the natural ones, in absence of such external intelligent agents, we shall admit that the interrelations emerge *spontaneously* among components and guided by some internal *purpose*. In either case, *intelligence* is involved in all associations that result in a new *identity*. The new identity is a creation of form and function, of a new being, instrument, or work of art. Intelligence and purpose must operate in the selection of the appropriate components and their relationships to crystallize a successful product. In other words, in any *natural spontaneous association* that results in an order, organization or pattern, the components have *intelligence* and *power of decision* to associate and they do it in a peculiar way.

Wills, intelligences, emotions and thoughts are accepted *realities* although not of the concrete type. They are set aside from scientific notice because they cannot be instrumentally detected. Still the force of their existence is compelling. Their dictates are powerful and unavoidable. These *intangibles realities* are precisely the fundamental ingredients of the unraveled puzzle of soul and mind, the architectural blocks of human culture and institutions, the core of human values and human evolvement. The ignorance of the *intangibles* in the inanimate world is even more acute for the same reason, their *undetectibility,* it shall be added that their effects are not so *immediately* obvious.

Physics is the exploration and questioning of physical action. If *identity* in the inanimate world *is connected to action* as happened in biosystems although in a more elementary way, it will be a monumental error to brush aside such *identity* from the field of physics. This thesis will make the case that the *identities* of inanimate things are responsible for the cosmic organization in the elemental and inanimate world.

Identities in living beings are highly distinctive although fragile and more dependent in *living interrelations* than in the material cells of their bodies. Life breeds a continuous turnover of elements and an interchange of resources with the outside. The *identity* of the living creature is preserved despite the total replacement of its material body. Not so when the *interrelations to the identity* collapse. Every body element remains intact, (it has been observed that some tissues as hair and nails continue growing for some time as separate formations) when *life of the creature* closes the door and stops its functions. Between life and death there is a critical bridge quickly crossed, in an instant, in which these *living interrelations* are irreversibly severed and the *identity* that *was* departs forever.

What are the nature of these relationships upon which rests the *identity* of the living creature? Are living-identities and living interrelations substantially different from non-living identities of the inanimate world? Or are they different degrees of expression of a unique reality? If so, what is the *fundamental* common denominator in the *identities* of living and non-living beings? We will attempt to answer these questions considered essential to physical reality and its operation. Identity in general deserves the attention of physics as potential *cause of action.*

7

IDENTITY OF NATURAL GROUPS. - ORDINARY AND ELEMENTAL PHYSICAL REALITY.

It is undeniable that *ordinary* reality confronts us with an abstract item undetectable by instrumentation, its *identity.* How shall we approach an inquiry about the *identity* of natural reality, which is *universally* present in each and such distinct things and creatures? In this study science makes us face two important problems: the inaccessibility of the elemental world and the lack of standard to evaluate the abstract.

Obviously the world of the smallest may express the abstraction of *identity* in its simplest terms, including its very existence. Thus, it appears that in an attempt to understand *identity*, these elemental items, the subatomic particles, should be the place to start our search. But unfortunately *it is not so* because in the world of the smallest, science tells us that matter and energy are *not accessible to precise measurement, location* and *observation.* Not because it is costly or difficult, but because it is *impossible!* Therefore, if precise knowledge of the *concrete* is impossible, less possible would be the knowledge of the *abstract* identity.

Let's turn to the physics of the microworld for explanations. The quantum theory postulates that matter and energy in their simplest form, photons, electrons, neutrons, protons and about another two hundred elemental particles (most of them artificially obtained and their life span very short of the order of one millionth of a second) appear as indivisible units, represented as wave-packets, and irreducible energy-packets named *quanta*. Recently these subatomic particles too have been found to have constituents named quarks. About one dozen of them have been detected.

Nature has a granular structure a concept more difficult to understand in the case of energy that we ordinarily envisioned as a continuous fluid. Not any more. For example, the energy of heat radiation is emitted discontinuously in *bundles* of specific frequencies, and energy associated to elemental particles also has *integral* values multiple of quanta. Even stranger to us, electrons, while rotating in their orbits, do that also *discontinuously* jumping from one position to another position which defines a new *quantified* energetic state, without leaving any trace in between these states. As if they actually dematerialize to materialize after again, in the new state. (Apparently each energetic state has its own *identity*. However at present we won't enter into this argument.) At the micro level both matter and energy are one and the same thing, interchangeable between each other. Matter can be converted into energy and energy into matter always preserving their *discontinuity*.

Quantum physics has further demonstrated that it is *theoretically* impossible to know with accuracy ultimate *concrete* reality. Beyond certain limits it cannot be determined with certainty the *position* of an elemental particle and the energy associated to it called *momentum* (momentum=mass x velocity), which reflects its state of motion. To determine the *position* of the particle inevitably carries an *uncertainty* in determining the value of its *momentum,* and vice versa. This uncertainty does not depend on the lack of precision of the instrumentation but is intrinsic to *the very nature* of physical reality. In other words, no matter how accurate the measurement or how sophisticated the instrumentation used, we will never be able to break this *uncertainty*. Matter and energy in the smallest dimensions are *immanently* elusive, unknowable. The mathematical expression of these limitations is given by the Heisenberg relation $\Delta\mathbf{M} \times \Delta\mathbf{V} \leq \mathbf{h}$ amply confirmed by experience (M stands for momentum, V for position and h is a constant). The knowledge of the *concrete* is hidden behind the Heisenberg threshold, separated from our perception by an unsurpassable, impenetrable wall that future technology will never cross. Consequently **if** the *concrete* cannot be perceived, assessed, valued with precision in the micro dimensions, certainly we must abandon the hope of obtaining any information about the *abstract* identity that *emanates from it* (as this

10

thesis will explore) and *manifestates throughout it* to sensorial observation and/or on physical action.

Excepting the micro-particles that are supposed to be the basic blocks and ultimate units of *concrete* reality, the rest of the creation are systems made up of the *association* of less complex ones. Consequently, it seems inescapable that *natural associations* and *the relationships between their components* shall be the first subject to study in order to understand *the essence and self-manifestation of physical reality*, the *identity* of things and creatures.

Another problem is how to handle the abstract in some sort of scientific terms when *exclusively* the focus of science is on the concrete. Thus, reality escapes scientific inquiry on two fronts: the microworld and the intangibles. The first due to the self-protected escape of nature expressed by Heisenberg's equation. The second by the self imposed limitations of science to ignore what is not instrumentally detectable.

Our search by necessity will need to abandon familiar scientific methods and adopt a primarily philosophical approach, thought experiments and mental models, reserving the empiric approach of observation and experiment for confirmation and application of the theory. This proceeding has already been advanced by physicists of the caliber of Professor Einstein.

We are used to interpret and reduce nature to mathematic equations. In the study of associations that will help but not a great deal because mathematical groups are extremely simple and inflexible compared with natural ones and fare poorly in accommodating these ones. Equations are built in one solely anonymous entity: *the number,* and number is a slim reflection of reality that besides not including the complications of nature also ignores its simplifications and shortcuts. Any formula, code or representation denudes physical reality of body and soul by eliminating some of the **concrete** and totally the **abstract**. A poet may decry that the song of the Creation is lost with such interpretation. The scientific methods to dissect, to focus, to analyze, to compartmentalize, would not unveil the *essence* of reality but would rather facilitate the escape of it. Plucking the petals of a rose is the very act that destroys the creature to be investigated, its *identity*, its *harmony*, its *beauty* and its *life*. Scientific theories are nothing else than *mental* constructs to explain *specific* events based on *some* aspects of reality; a straight line of limitations. This theory, aware of its limitations, is a mere step to address the *universal* and *total* with the expectation to initiate and facilitate similar workings, and develop useful applications.

IDENTITY, THE UNIVERSAL QUESTION.

Reality is perceived as separate unities with an indivisible, unseverable, intransferible *identity*. Should this identity not be an intrinsic *essence* of reality as well as its external manifestation the entire Creation would be a deceitful devise for its own creatures. The basic foundations of reality, the *identities* shall be common texture to all things and creatures rather than sporadic features subject to fundamental changes -as that of its very existence- along the cosmos or processes of evolution. No scientific thought could be conceived on a universe inconsistent with itself where part of it could be identifiable and part not, as it would be the situation if each and every thing and creature could not claim its *identity*. Because of this *universality*, identities are *essences* of reality.

Elemental particles and quanta of energy, despite our inability to perceive them with precision, ought to be *identifiable* independent entities should the quantum barrier to their perception be removed. Two reasons come to mind. One is that while new identities appear in the process of association, the identities of the components are consistently preserved in every association as it can be checked in the reverse process of division. The only *identity* **lost** in the division -and

13

logically so because the system is destroyed– is *that of
the divided system*. (I emphasize the word <u>lost</u> because
I firmly believe that *the abstract* once created cannot
be destroyed by concrete means. There is no hammer to
crash a thought). *Unseparated* components conserve their
identity in the association as well as when dislocated
from it. There is no indication to support a change of
rules in the *ultimate division* of physical reality. The
second reason is that *separated* elemental particles
must have *identities* when such *identities* are needed to
organize and be recognized in the organization of the
association.

With the contribution of the information theories
it seems no longer acceptable to avoid the *abstract,*
the *identity*, in the study of physical reality. It is
embodied on it. Identity is *the universal question* in the
understanding of the universe, including us. *Identity*
may well be a flag under which are hidden other *essential
features* of reality that trigger phenomena.

Because ordinary reality –the solely detectable–
are *groupings* of others down the line to the ultimate
units of matter and energy, it is clear that the study
of *association* should start with finding answers about
identity. New identities emerge at every step in the
process of association. What *drives* lead to association?
What are the *standards* to select components? Where are
the fundamental forces of *order and organization* rooted?

What *causes* the control of an association? Eventually answers to these features of *association* would lead to those pertaining to *universal* features of *identity* and physical reality.

Has *identity* a role in the process of association? Are other *universal* characters entwined with *identity* and its possible operation on physical reality? How is *identity* connected to the principle of life? Are living creatures a type of reality *essentially* different from the rest of natural realities? Are there some consistent principles guiding the evolution of living beings to man and that of elemental particles to every other system? The process of *association* poses basic questions and answers to them, verification and utilization of such findings are at the aims of this theory of systems, identity and cosmic evolution.

CHAPTER II. - FIRST POSTULATE OF THIS THEORY OF NATURAL SYSTEMS.

We are acquainted with the phenomenon of *selective intelligent decision* in complex systems like creatures. This subject will now be placed under scrutiny in regard to the elemental level of matter-energy.

The **first postulate** of this thesis is that **elemental matter-energy has an elemental capability to make decisions and meaning out of information.**

That is, the *selective intelligent decisions* we observe in creatures are in a most rudimentary degree rooted in the initial particles of the Creation. If the word *decision* and *meaning* are objectionable to the reader because they are associated with highly developed creatures, *pre-acting energy* instead of decision and *awarded-perception* instead of intelligence can substitute them. The former standing for the capacity to trigger action and the latter for the faculty to draw self-significance from information. We go to explore if these capacities would reveal themselves in an imaginary binding of two indivisible elements A and B located in a universe of similar elements. The term **information** is here taken in its broadest sense, meaning any reality identifiable to the observer, element or system, in question.

Let us define **meaningful relationship** between an energetic element A and another B as a bond, whatever its nature, that contains information from A and from B, the **meaning** of which is interpreted, restricted and acceptable to elements A and B respectively. The significance that the information may have for A and for B is not necessarily the same.

If the bond is a *form of energy* supplied by A and B, which are the sole source of the bond, it must be a *fraction* of the energies of A and B. No elements give their total energy when binding. It would be annihilation instead of binding, and no bond is possible without elements to bind.

The bond shall have some *permanence* otherwise the relation between both elements is collision rather than binding. When two natural elemental entities represented by A and B *relate* among themselves with certain permanency and *do not relate to others* that are equally qualified, the binding is supposed to be a *selective action.* It implies that the elements:

1) have an **inherent power to decide** to bind, a faculty of choice, or a pre-acting energy that guides action, and

2) have an **inherent awareness of the meaning** that the bond AB would have to each one.

The question at hand is: Whether **real elemental matter** represented by A and B is capable to make *selective decisions,* that is, *controls* its actions and knows the *meaning* of information. Such capabilities shall manifest in the process of binding A and B.

The *inherent* control or power to decide, here referred, shall not be confused with *forced* control. The first is an *essential* feature of the *identity.* The second is an *external pressure upon the identity* and not embodied in it. The difference was illustrated in the Introduction of this Thesis with the example of a prisoner. He has at all times control of his power to decide, his free decision, although he might not enjoy the benefits or results of it because chains restrain him. Freedom of decision is an *essential* faculty of the prisoner, inherent and intransferable. While the chain, a *forced* control, is a restrain upon his movements but not upon his volition that is always free. The chain can be removed and transferred to another prisoner without detriment of the essential characters of either one.

Let's consider the possible circumstances under which bond AB might occur assuming that the agencies of *decision* and *meaning; 1)* be vested in A and B *which represent elemental matter*, 2) not vested in A and B but vested in outside entities, or 3) not vested in any element at all, that is, non existing. The number of possible situations is nine.

There are only three situations with regard to power of decision.

SITUATION No. 1. - *Power of decision* is vested in A and B respectively.

SITUATION No. 2. - *Power of decision* is vested in outsiders.

SITUATION No. 3. - *Power of decision* is not vested in A, in B, or in outsiders.

Still in each of these situations the capability to make *meaning of information* can be vested: 1) in A and in B, 2) in outsiders, or 3) in none of them. That raises the number of possible situations to nine.

CHART No. 1 frames the nine possibilities.

CHART No. 1

SITUATION	DECISION	MEANING
1)	in A and in B not in outsiders	a) in A, in B, not in outsiders b) not in A, not in B, <u>but</u> in outsiders (X) c) not in A, not in B, not in outsiders
2)	not in A, not in B in outsiders	a) in A, in B, not in outsiders b) not in A, not in B, <u>but</u> in outsiders (XX) c) not in A, not in B, not in outsiders
3)	not in A, not in B not in outsiders	a) in A, in B, not in outsiders b) not in A, not in B, <u>but</u> in outsiders (XXX) c) not in A, not in B, not in outsiders .

The following discussion shows that **binding** is only possible in <u>SITUATION 1a)</u> where A and B are the only elements capable to make *decisions* and *meaning* out of information about their bonding. And as binding of elements has occurred since the Big Bang and ever after the **first postulate of this thesis shall be taken as proven.**

In **SITUATION 1b)** the elements A and B *decide* but they are impermeable to their mutual information that somehow spills to the outside and the outsiders are able to interpret it for A and for B (See X). We face here the absurdity that the **informed** (outsiders) ca*nnot decide*, while the **uninformed** (A and B) blindly *decide*. The conclusion, by generalizing this action to the rest of the elements of the universe, is that the *intelligent* elements of it are *paralyzed observers* of the ignorant ones' activity. And those who play the game don't know how to play it.

But more irrational yet. The *intelligent* (informed) elements who understand the information of A and B will become *ignorant* (uninformed) *when making their own binding,* for as said, they decide their binding but do not understand its *meaning*. How then do the *intelligent* elements **lose** the capability to **make meaning** out of information on their *own affairs* when they were able to meaningfully conduct the *affairs of others*?

The opposite would happen to A and B, that by being *ignorant* of the meaning of their own binding suddenly they will become *intelligent* to understand the others' binding when the occasion arises. There is no way to explain this **changing on-off** in the faculty to make *meaning* of information. More so because it is more difficult to understand others than themselves. And more *unproportionate* yet to understand the bindings of *many other elements of the universe* and not the *single one* between themselves.

This situation is unacceptable to reason.

In SITUATION 1c) the elements A and B *decide* but no element in the entire creation including A and B understand the *meaning* of the information upon which the decision is made. There is no intelligent basis for the decision. Elements A and B and by extension all elements decide in complete blindness.

Now the question arises: How and at *what point* of evolution do the highly evolved systems as *creatures acquire the capacity to make meaning* of information? Leaving without answer the "how" (because no explanation is possible), *that point* would have marked the reversal from *unpurposeful action* in that part of the universe to a *purposeful* one, still leaving the **unevolved** contemporary systems as well as simpler components of the *evolved ones* **without purpose.** The acquisition of such capacity in a universe deprived of it at the elemental level, would require a miracle. Not a simple miracle but a complex one according to the complexity of the system in question. And many of them, for the appearance of every system able to benefit from information would be a new miracle. Thus, the number of them would exceed the human population of all times, assuming that we include other biosystems. Therefore, this Situation 1c) is unsustainable under the light of reason, or faith.

To deny to the binding elements A and B the capacity to make *meaning* of information on their bindings – SITUATIONS 1b), 1c) - is, in principle, the denial of order, organization, hierarchy and evolution. Harmonies don't occur without intelligence for they are based in order and order comes from: 1) understood compromises *among parties,* 2) organization from *intelligent* coordination of processes, 3) hierarchy from structuration of *intelligent* powers, and 4) evolution from the evolvement of those capacities and controls by a *rational process*. (Fundamental **principles** of elemental reality and **process of evolvement** are missed in our present view of the universe). And as order, organization, hierarchy and evolution are present at all levels, this SITUATION 1c) is flatly defeated by overwhelming empirical data.

In SITUATION 2a) A and B are *intelligent* elements able to draw *meaning* from the elementary information conveyed to and from each other. But they have not *the capability to make decisions* on their own. Outsiders, not knowing the *significance* that the bond AB has for A and B, decide for them to bind; and viceversa A and B decide the bindings of outsiders, presumably many of them, without knowing the meaning of such bindings.

If the cause of binding A and B is *decided* by *uninformed* outsiders, the next questions are: How does **matter** outside of A and B have the power to decide -*arbitrarily (in ignorance)*- while A and B - **same matter** also- cannot decide *intelligently its own binding?* Has nature granted *power of decision* to matter in *unintelligent status* while denying such power of decision to matter in *intelligent status*? The awareness of information would be *useless* because decisions are not made <u>upon</u> it. Thus, such awareness should not appear in nature or should have disappeared long ago for lack of exercise since the Big Bang occurred.

The phenomenon of binding cannot be split and inconsequential: one party knows the significance of the bond, another *ignorant* party decides. That conflicts with conceptual and experimental logic. Elements A and B would be at the mercy of *chance (uninformed)* for they are crippled *not in their intelligence* but in their capacities to *decide.*

The absurdity of previous SITUATION 1b) is being repeated in this SITUATION 2a): those that don't know how to play, play the game. Plus, this situation implies that outsiders would lose the power of *decision* when making their own bonds. Again the irrational switch on-off of faculties, in this case the power of decision. By what process power of *decision* would be lost or acquired? There are no rational answers, therefore SITUATION 2a) is unsustainable.

In <u>SITUATION 2b)</u> outsiders have both power to *decide* for A and B and to make *meaning* of information while A and B have neither (See XX). The questions now are: How outsiders to A and B have the power to decide and to make meaning of information for A and B while A and B have not these faculties despite being elemental **matter**

also, and precisely the *ones interested in the binding?* If this was the case the initial universe would had *misplaced such faculties* from the interested parties to the uninterested ones. And again we face the switch on-off absurdity: The outside matter will not draw meaning on its own bondings, nor will decide its own binding while having both capacities for alien ones. No explanation can be given to these suppositions and thus SITUATION 2b) is unacceptable.

In <u>SITUATION 2c)</u> outsiders *decide* not understanding the information conveyed between A and B which are also ignorant elements. Now, *all elements are ignorant, deciding for others, but unable to decide for themselves.* Here both absurdities are combined; one, the switch on-off effect on the power of decision, and two, the misplacement of *power of decision* from the parties interested in the binding (A and B) to the uninterested ones (the outsiders).

The consequences along evolution further defy this situation. Outsiders having **inherent** control over these two elements A and B would also control the rest of the elements conjoining A and B in the making of a system, if ever an intelligent system could have been developed by totally unintelligent matter! The resulting system would be controlled by the outsiders instead of having *inherent* control of its own organization. This is repugnant to reason and contrary to evidence in highly developed systems as living creatures. The universe would have no evolutionary intelligent direction whatsoever if this *Situation 2c)* were valid. It would be populated by *indecisive* (in their own affairs) elements and systems **without purpose** because **no one** including outsiders understood information. **Binding** would take place **by chance (uninformed)**, blind bonds in total absence of intelligence, logic or reason.

Objecting that outsiders may be under intelligent controls of others does not solve the problem, it *transfers it* to another controller. Escalating the transfer, who would ultimately make *intelligent* decisions for all elemental particles, and, at all times? Where are these controllers if not in the universe?

This Situation translates into two extreme contradictions: An amazingly *active universe* made up of *passive* matter-energy incapable to decide their own actions and too *ignorant* to understand them.

In SITUATION 3a) the action of the universe is *not decided* by any element, although every one is able to interpret information *in their own bonding.* But they cannot use it because they cannot decide. As already said, being A and B awareness of information of no use, it shall not appear in nature or shall disappear for lack of exercise. Nature eliminates the unnecessary and the faculty to make meaning out of information that *cannot be used* would be a waste of universal proportions: *A universe of intelligent matter incapable to decide.* Furthermore, matter will be crippled in its *abstract faculties* by having intelligence (abstract) but no power of decision (abstract). This half concession of abstract faculties is self-defeated and enough to eliminate SITUATION 3a) as an unacceptable half way compromise.

In SITUATION 3b) nobody *decides* (as in previous Situation) despite that outsiders can make meaning of the AB bond. Such awareness of information is useless again for bindings take place without deciders for even *chance* shall be *out of the universe* because *it is an intelligent one* and *chance* is not.(See XXX). Notice that *chance* is merely a fiction in substitution for the unanswered. This word shall be eliminated from the scientific literature.

The Situation 3b) is even more absurd than the previous one because it adds the *switch on-off* effect in the *elemental intelligence* of the entire universe. Matter is intelligent for others but not for itself. Where does such intelligence **goes** when it is switched off in the process of its own binding? The Situation 3b does not resist scrutiny nor do any theory of physical reality based on these premises.

In SITUATION 3c) we have an *ignorant* and *indecisive* universe of elemental matter and energy *ruled by chance*. This, by the way, is our present scientific stance!

Here the *switch on-off* effect does not appear at the elemental level as happened in Situations 1, 2a, 2b, 2c, and 3b, but the unexpected in spectacular dimensions happens during evolution. *These faculties* **appear** *and not in the primitive form that corresponds to* **elemental** *matter but in the specific form fit to each and every living creature.*

If the *switch on-off* effect was not absurd enough in the elemental world, as already described, here it **suddenly operates in great variety and** in *highly evolved form*. How these faculties appear **without seeds in elemental matter** nor **process of evolvement** is a mystery. More so when the **components** of creatures **remain without such faculties** as scientific notions have it. Only the integral being will have them!

The Situation 3c) proposition actually establishes a miracle trade of phenomenal proportions. Highly evolved faculties had appeared again and again in the past and still more evolved ones are to be expected in the future. Our knowledge of evolution guarantees it! Situation 3c) brings us to an incalculable number of surprising wonders. We don't need continuous and unending miracles to remind us that the Creation is a miracle. But only, one single one: its coming into existence **as it is.**

POWER OF DECISION AND FACULTY TO MAKE MEANING OUT OF INFORMATION ARE ESSENTIAL ATTRIBUTES OF THE UNIVERSE.

POWER OF DECISION. – It shall be accepted that A and B can decide for themselves and their bindings for the opposite leads to the unacceptable conclusion of the need of **compelling controllers** in every action of the elemental quanta of physical reality. If such controllers are in this universe, the power of decision has been misplaced on them rather than to be placed in the parties interested in the action, both *equally qualified matter*. If the controllers cannot be found around, then the universe is inconsistent with itself for the causes of its functioning are *out of it.*

Such *controller or controllers* ruling a universe that is indecisive had later in evolution delegated the power to decide -in a most evolved form- to living creatures. By what process this delegation or creation of *power of decision* took place? It is impossible to answer this question if *power of decision* is not attributed to **elemental** matter, in **elementary** form and found in a rational **process of evolvement of such power of decision** in nature.

Without an **evolvement process** of the power of decision from an **elementary form** to that of superior systems only miracles will justify our Creation. For such Creation

a)   would have been defectively planned in not giving power of decision to elemental matter,

b)   would have made amendments by giving it to living creatures,

c)   would continue to be defective in the non-living world and

d)   would expect successive miracles to fill up future evolutionary vacuums.

The Creation, **as it is**, is the sole miracle admissible on **its own evidence** and so it is the **inherent power of elemental matter to make decisions** for reduction at the absurd.

FACULTY TO MAKE MEANING OUT OF INFORMATION. – The faculty to make *meaning* of information (Situation 1a) shall be accepted together with the power of decision in the entire universe or we will run into the absurdities discussed in Situations 1b, 1c, 2a, 2b, 2c, 3a, 3b, and 3c.

It can be repeated the said in Situation 1c), that the negation of an **elementary** capacity to make *meaning* of information is, in principle, the denial of order, organization, hierarchy and evolution. It is contrary to experience in highly developed systems, and contrary to the internal meaningful regulation of the microworld whether being or not being component of higher systems.

Thus, we must conclude that **SITUATION 1a)** is the only one rational and possible for all matter-energy. In addition, it is *essentially* necessary for the uniformity of the universe and the consistency of any theory about it and its evolution.

Going back to the definition of *meaningful relationships*, it shall be clarified the last sentence: "acceptable to A and B". Logically when one element decides, it must have some basis for the decision. It can be expected that the bond AB will be accomplished **if** it is acceptable to A and B. *Spontaneous relations* would become stable equilibrium when *mutual good* for the interrelated parties results, and statistically it would be the case among *intelligent* elements. Harmonic equilibrium will be the result.

SECOND POSTULATE OF THIS THEORY.

Second postulate of this thesis: **The pre-acting energy or power of elemental matter-energy to decide is the ultimate variable of elemental physical reality.** This postulate is obvious by definition of terms.

Experience tells us that errors of action, that is, rejection of an intelligent improvement, a convenient *bond,* occur. Error is not an occurrence exclusive to man. It happens at every level of matter and systems of the universe. It is the prerogative of *decision* when it is free, independent from any other variable. In short, when power to *decide* is the *ultimate variable* of physical reality, which hereof is postulated. The different evolutionary rates, the variety of things and creatures in the universe, the unequal distribution of matter-energy, and ultimately the free will of man are extensive confirmations of this postulate.

The ultimate support to this postulate is given by the quantum theory and quantum experiments. Precisely the quantum theory was originated by the unexpected behavior of elemental particles breaking the laws of Classic Physics. Not only do they break the law but also no law could predict the **individual** behavior of these particles. The reason is and could not be other than the **elemental particles have free will.**

CHAPTER III. - SYSTEMS AND RELATIONS.

This Chapter will dwell in the structure of physical reality. Except for the elemental matter most of physical reality appears in associations that will be characterized as **natural systems.**

To define is always a difficult task, more so in the present theory where we shall define **natural system** when that is the very subject to be studied and whose most fundamental essence, its *identity*, is an abstract philosophical item not a scientific one. Abstract realities have been ignored due to the empirical approach of science that relies only on the accidental and descriptive.

Another difficulty arises from the fact that systems frequently have the double role of *system* and *component* of another system. Actually all systems have this dual role if the universe is considered to be a system.

A preliminary definition could be to state that a **natural system** is **an _identifiable_ being or reality,** clearly _distinct from its constituents_ **that are linked by _meaningful relationships._**

These statements convey three requirements to qualify as a system:

1) The system has an *identity*, the manifestation of self. We accept the identity of creatures and ordinary things in their own evidence. Each is a being distinct from others.

2) The system is built upon components and although these cause its existence the system is *clearly distinct* from them.

3) The components and the system are *meaningfully related* among themselves. The surroundings and external relations are not part of the system because they are *not direct and immanent cause of it or of its organization.*

Postulates and conclusions of this thesis will apply equally to *all systems* whatever they might be, universe or creature, living being or inanimate matter, whole or components.

In my attempted definition I interposed the phrase **clearly distinct from its constituents** to emphasize that the *identity* is the *fundamental feature* of the system. In man, for instance, identity is equated not much to material elements, chemical reactions and physical relations, as to the abstract texture of his personality which is *permanent* regardless of the transformations or status of his body. Concrete elements, in fact, are continuously being substituted by other ones without impairing the *identity* of the man.

Whereas *identifying* creatures is not a problem, with other systems there is ample room for confusion especially if they are not of ordinary dimensions or if one is a component of another. Such systems shall be specifically described when referring to them.

We also run into problems with *interrelations* because in systems integrated by less complex ones their interrelations overstep one another. For example, the universe qualifies as a system. It is a unique structure emerging as a *single whole, nothing is unrelated within it* and *beyond it no physical reality is known*. It stays by itself. However, the relations among the constituents of the universe may be an obstacle to determine the interrelations of a system in the universe and setting them apart from those of the universe. The same accounts for bodies of living creatures that are made up of cells, themselves intricate worlds of interrelations. Cells are *real* systems as well as components of the body and the internal relations of the body, except for those within the organization of the cell itself, shall be considered external and unrelated to the cell-system.

Maria L. Costell Gaydos

Immediately after the Big Bang there were not many *types of relations* among the initial components. The universe was an uncomplicated system. This simple situation did not last too long for soon *new relations* appeared in celestial formations building diverse organizations and frontiers and defining new systems: galaxies, planets, stars, etc., These *relations* besides holding together each of the new systems were also the ones that originated the different *identities* of those systems. New *physical realities, new systems,* were created in spectacular measure. What we may call cosmic evolution or evolution of the universe, was and properly is the *process of creation of systems* and *identities.*

The importance of *relations* in a system derives from the fact that they enjoy some kind of stability and shield a territory that legitimizes the existence and identity of the new system. Transient events or collisions vanish without significance. Instead *system's interrelations* provide both *pattern* and *durability,* the basic features of **order** and **organization, of its own order and organization.** No transient situation allows for prediction and application of any knowledge of it because the situation will never repeat itself at another time. What characterizes disorder is total unpredictability; no law can be deduced from it. Systems on the contrary are *displays of order and pattern.* Their very existence conveys *useful* information to outsiders.

36

They are **information** and upon such information further order and organization can be created.

As time progressed, a variety and proliferation of **relations** emerged in novel orders and structures, in and out of systems, and although diversity and complexity increased *order prevailed in the entire universe.*

Granted that order results from systems' inter*relations* and that evolvement of order leads to *organization* let's now illustrate that the **drive to organize** is a natural occurrence **innate to matter.** Concrete reality evolved into systems since the beginning of the Creation by its own internal resources, a *spontaneous* metamorphosis that we continuously see on this planet and beyond it.

It has been observed that certain crystals undergo spectacular changes of structure when passing through various intervals of temperatures. Neither temperature nor heat is endowed with any faculty *to organize or reorganize crystal lattices.* Such faculty is obviously invested *on matter* and sparkling **in concert** from each particle of the crystal.

Natural production of coacervates, macrospheres, membranes or simple organic matter are sure samples of matter **spontaneous self-organization** in absence of external controllers with knowledge in such affairs. No less spontaneous is the emerging of atoms from elemental particles, of molecules from atoms, or planetary systems from explosions of stellar bodies. The initial universe took an *incredible short time* to show its colossal means of self-organization. The power of matter to create order and organization cannot be dismissed. It takes place in all spaces, at all times, a course that starting with elemental Hydrogen incessantly claimed up to the creation of all physical reality, as we know it. It is the continuous trend of physical reality, intrinsic to matter rather than imposed.

All that said, it is clear that the power of organization derives logically from what is postulated by this thesis for organization implies *meaningful interrelations* that are based on *intelligent* components able to *decide* (See First and Second Postulate of this thesis in previous chapter). However, interrelations will occur only if elemental matter has **a drive to associate** with other elements. That brings us to the third postulate of this thesis.

THIRD POSTULATE OF THIS THEORY OF NATURAL SYSTEMS.
Elemental matter and energy is essentially endowed with a social drive to interrelate.

The *unassociated* matter populating the cosmic spaces expresses not the lack of social drive but the paramount fact that *freedom of decision is inviolable*. Physical reality is free to decide the use of any of its capacities including its intelligence and essential urges.

Another phenomenon that this theory will explain and becomes patent in the building of organization and simultaneous to it, is that of the production of **external control (forced control)**. The integration of a system depends on **internal controls** that transcend into **external control** without which its existence would collapse. It is undeniable that organized matter can exert a *forced* control in non- or less- organized matter. Higher organizations have more efficient controls than lower ones. The degree of a system's *external control* is directly related to its *complexity and intelligence*. Living creatures use their environments to obtain food, energy, joy, information and means of reproduction. These wonders are possible throughout the high level of clever arrangements and efficient regulations of biosystems. We will see next that the roots of *external*

39

control shall be found in the evolvement of systems far before living creatures exerted such external control.

GENESIS OF SYSTEMS. - PRELIMINARY CRITICAL NUMBER.

A minimum number of elements are needed to build a system. To construct a table you must have four pieces: a top and at least three legs to support the top. Two legs are insufficient while there is no limit to the number of legs that a table sufficiently large might have.

Natural occurring systems emerge **not** before a minimum number of components have been reached. We will name this number: **critical number** Nc.

Let's consider an imaginary aggregation of indivisible energetic elements A, B, C, D, etc., that comply with these conditions:

a)   All the elements of the group have the same amount of energy.

b)   Each element is related to all others, and each pair of elements shares a single bond or relation.

c)   All bonds carry the same amount of energy independently of direction, shape or trajectory of the bond. (This assumption is based on the grounds that our aggregation, although it has observable dimensions, is integrated by elemental particles with speeds close to the speed of light. These particles enclosed in ordinary systems will sweep its internal distances in a fraction of a second. Ordinary distances are irrelevant for the elementary world).

d)   Each element contributes equal energy to the bond, named **Ex** (for external energy), and remains with an internal energy **Ei** (for internal energy). Naming **Et** the total energy of the elements before binding, it can be establish that **Et = Ex + Ei**.

This simplistic imaginary model is far from being a *physical reality* but, as we will see later, the deductions made upon it are valid for **all systems** and the simplifications here adopted further support the final conclusions deduced.

Take a series of aggregations (as defined above) each having **one** elemental **unit** more than the previous group. Starting with the first group of two elements, the next will have three, the following four, etc. We bring to a graph *the sum of energies of each group's elements* (in OY coordinates) versus *the number of elements of the group* (on OX coordinates) **Figure No. 1.**

Assuming that each element has energy OP, the first system's energy (2 elements) shall be represented by point Q in which: OQ = 2OP. The next group's energy (3 elements) will be point K being OK = 3OP. The points of every group's energy will fall in the straight line OT.

This is an *upper limit approximation* because a fraction of the energy goes in the binding and consequently the line should be likely curved as OT'.

The sum of the bonds' energy in each system shall produce a line similar to OG starting on S if the energy carried by a single bond is OS. The line OG is parabolic due to the fact that the number of relations increases at an accelerated pace while the elements on the groups increase one by one.

The formula for the number of interrelations is N(N-1)/2 for each element relates to N-1 others and does not relate to itself. The total number shall be divided by 2 for every relation has been counted twice. The AB relation was counted from A to B and later from B to A . Bringing the numbers of **Table No. 1** to the graph, we make an interesting finding. No matter how small the energy of interrelations could be, *after a sufficient number of elements,* the two lines will cross at a point C, which correspond to a number of elements which we will name **Nc** for **critical number.**

Critical number Nc indicates **the number of elements for which the sum of the bonds' energy is equal to the sum of the elements' energy**. A group with a number of elements greater than **Nc** will have a net of interrelations with energy superior to that of all combined elements considering that the bonds are stable. **It is obvious that this is not possible if the group is not able to**

control and obtain energy from outside of the system.
(**Figure No. 1**). The alternative to obtain energy by
annihilation of some element to support the bonds' would
be self-defeated as the element eliminated is part of
one of the bonds already created. Its elimination would
cripple the bond. Therefore, **if the aggregation exceeds
the critical number <u>Nc</u> it must obtain energy from
outside, it must develop control of external energy, a
new power absolutely needed to its existence.**

We will arrive to the same two lines if we consider
a single group of two elements and we place them in a
box [**BOX-A**] adding new elements one by one, while taking
each time note of the total energies of the elements
and total energy of the bonds. What happens in the box
when Nc is reached? A balance of power among *elements*
and *bonds* is reached. The next element added to the box
will deliver the energetic power to the interrelations
according to the dynamics of the graph. **<u>Nc</u>** is the
critical number of change. Previous to **<u>Nc</u>,** the elements
ruled in the group, after **<u>Nc</u>** the bonds **will rule** in the
group and **the system will acquire control of external
energy. This is a typical power of systems and, in
general, of order and organization.**

A more dramatic view can be given with a scale.
Placing weights representing the elements' energy on
one plate and those representing the bonds' energy on
the other, one element more or less than **<u>Nc</u>** translates

---

in tilting a different plate. If the plate tilted is that of the bonds' energy the aggregation or system will acquire *control of external energy* needed to support the bonds. Should the elements and bonds within the group disagree -so to speak- the stronger, *the bonds, would impose control over the others*. But such discord unlikely shall occur, for the *bonds* are **tacit** *accords* among elements, and harmony will reign.

ENERGY-CONTROL. - SUBORDINATION. - HIERARCHY.

Is it the same **type** of energy that of the elements **A, B, C,** . etc., and that of the bonds they originate? Or is it a **qualitative** distinction between these energies? (The term **type** refers to the **essential** characters of the energy, that is, of the physical reality.)

Real elemental particles are supposed to be indivisible. They have no parts, therefore no attachments to link parts either. Thus when they interrelate as in chemical compounding the bond (the valence) is interpreted as two electrons circling in a common trajectory between the atoms. The undivided electrons make up the bond by their *temporary* presence in every point of the trajectory. Equally in our imaginary system the elemental units cannot be divided. The bond **AB** shall be interpreted as a *temporal* sharing of the energetic units **A** and **B** back and forth to their original provinces.

44

Mathematical formulations treat energy as an *amorph* quantity independent of the path or origin of the energy or its *content of information.* According to this approach the *bonds' energy* will be merely *the sum of the* ***A*** *and* ***B*** *energetic contributions to it*, and if several elements contributed to a relationship similarly the sum of their quantitative contributions. However, because this thesis postulates that elemental matter-energy is endowed with capacity to *make decisions* and *meaning out of information*, the situation of a real event is entirely different.

Since the binding of elemental matter **A** and **B** is a sharing of these **same** undivided elements the bond **AB** is the **same type** (referring to their **essential** features) of energy of **A** and **B** and consequently shall carry too the *capacity to make decisions and meaning out of information*. Plus these capacities would be *qualitative and quantitative superior* to the capacities of **A** and **B** for they deal not with a single unit **A** or **B** but with both **A** and **B** as we shall see now.

A decision made by the bond **AB** decides for **A** and for **B.** Such deed (to decide for **A** and for **B**) neither single element **A** or **B** has the capacity to do. Each decides exclusively for itself. Then in terms of *quantitative control,* the bond's energy is superior to each of the **A** and **B** energies for its *decisions subordinate two elements instead of one.*

45

The *increase of power* when *information increases* (observable in natural systems) is easy to explain with our imaginary model assigning, as this theory does, a *qualitative* aspect to the energy as follows: If elements **A**, **B** and **C** have different content of information but equal quantity of energy a bond AB will decide for **A** and for **B** but not for **C**. Not only because **C** is not contained in the system but because the bond **AB** lacks the *inherent powers to interpret C's information* which is not contained in bond **AB**. While bond **AC** will decide for **A** and **C** but not for **B** for the same reasons. In other words, bond **AC** is an energy alien, external to **B**, that can only exert a *force control* upon **B**, not an *intelligent one.*

There is a **qualitative** distinction between the bonds **AB** and **AC** despite both having the same quantity of energy. Their *inherent decisions* are based on their *content of information*. Thus energy has a *qualitative* aspect based on its informational content. It has an **inherent control** (I repeat not to be confused with *forced control*) upon *solely* its energetic **informational content**. Its content of information gives the energy its **qualitative aspect** that determines when its decisions are *voluntary* or *forced* controls.

Meaning being the significance that a system makes of a set of information depends on the type and amount of such information. The bond **AB** receives information from **A** and from **B** therefore containing information of both. It has more information than either element. It has evolved a power to make *meaning of more complex information and to make decisions for more information.* Its **decision,** just for being better informed, is **more powerful.** That is, information imparts power, **inherent control. Inherent control** cannot be attributed to the present notion of amorph energy considered *unrelated to information.*

Upon these new concepts this thesis will find it appropriate to change the conventional name of **energy** for a new name **control-energy. This** better reflects both the **quantitative** and the **qualitative** aspects of the energy when taken into consideration its *quantity* and its specific *content of information.*

Summarizing:

1.   When the number of the system's elements is superior to **Nc,** *the energy of the interrelations exceeds the total energy of the elements combined,* assuming that energy is amorph. Therefore, **the interrelations control the elements.**

2.   To support interrelations the system must exert *external control of energy* (forced control) upon other elements or systems alien to its intrinsic control (that may explain the need of living systems to obtain energy by breathing, eating, etc., for survival.)

3. The interrelations *control* elements and bonds on the basis of their amount of energy and *specific information.*

4. Systems confronting and competing with others *for external control* of energy must assert a hierarchic rank of *forced* energy. We may say that *external control* among systems is related – according to the new concept of *control energy*– to both the quantitative and qualitative aspects of their energies.

PYRAMIDS OF BONDS' ENERGIES.

Let's go back to our imaginary model in **BOX A.** By adding new elements to the aggregation after **Nc** had been reached, the number of interrelations increases at such an accelerated rate that soon the lines representing them overlap their nets becoming obscured by the heavy density of lines. No design that reflects the events will be feasible. (**Fig. No. 2**).

If *elemental energetic units* **relate**, why not the *bonds* which are also **energies,** and furthermore located in a more crowded situation with more occasions and better access to social relations? Certainly they should, and that would result in a new round of bonds each containing *information* from the two initial bonds that originate it. That is, *information from a total of* *four elements.* These bonds should be more powerful and able to *control the bonds* they linked, and the *elements* contained in these bonds.

These second round of bonds also intertwine among them creating new relations, new bonds, that will continue their inter-biding even *more actively* because the **number of bonds** that originated them (the second round bonds) **is superior to the number of the previous ones** (the first round of bonds), the environment is more crowded, the encounters more frequent. The production of successive bonds would escalate increasingly faster and easier because the successive conditions will be ever more favorable. Finally a *supreme stage of binding* will produce the **ultimate round of bonds** containing the *maximum information of the system,* all elements participating in each of these bonds. No subsequent bondings with new elements will be possible.

Perhaps by now we can graphically represent these **bonds' control-energies** in escalating strata within *upside down* pyramids with apexes enclaved in each of the in pyramidal bases to culminate in **the greatest bases,** consisting of **control-energies sharing energies of all elements of the aggregation.**

TOTAL CONTROL-ENERGY OF SYSTEMS: THE WILL.

Each of these **ultimate bonds** should be *quantitatively* and *qualitatively* powerful enough to subdue every element of the system for they contain all of them. But in addition, these **ultimate bonds** having *identical informational* content presumably will interrelate with no alternative left but to fuse into a *single total control-energy* of magnified intensity where the elemental powers and control-energies will become engulfed in ONE united control: the **WILL** of the system. By its own constitution this *unified energy control* will have the capacity to control the whole aggregation of elements and bonds at all times. And such **total control-energy** should be extraordinarily powerful in relation to the rest of the bonds and elements because now we are not dealing with the *control-energy of one single* bond -even the more powerful one- but with the **integration** of all the **ultimate bonds** which are the most numerous, best informed and loaded with the greatest amount of energy. A grandiose resonant effect!

The **WILL** by all means will control the system!

The **WILL** of living beings is the equivalent of the **total control-energy of the systems** in the rest of the physical reality.

ACTUAL CRITICAL NUMBER.

In defining **Nc** we considered the elemental units and their immediate bindings thus resulting the graph of **Fig. No. 1.** It can be seen that the **actual number** of relations is far greater than the number plotted in the graph that considers only the first round of bonds. The lines of the graph will cross much sooner by taking into account the number and energy of all interrelations which are greater than the number and energy of the first round bonds alone. Thus, the **actual critical number Nt** is far smaller than **Nc,** the preliminary one. Now **Nc** shall be disregarded as a crude approximation in our starting deductions. The **actual critical number Nt** is the **one** that marks the **creation** of a **new order, a system.**

Based only in *quantitative* considerations an aggregation having reached **Nt** number of elements is a **system** and acts as a whole, *an identity,* with unified **total control-energy** able to decide the fate of itself. This **integral control** defines the main operational character of a system. The crystal lattices that change organization at certain levels of temperature do so by **WILL,** the **total control-energy** created by their initial elements and their bondages. **WILL** will dominate elements and bondages at light speed, practically at once when translated to the crystal dimensions.

In addition the system inexorably needs to exercise *external control* to maintain *internal control* and its very existence. *The capacity of external control is ingrained in organized structures.*

Thus this theory provides a possible and logical description of:

1)   the formation of systems,

2)   the *energy-control* for their functioning,

3)   the systems' need to control *external energy* and

4)   the evolvement of the **WILL** of the systems.

POTENTIAL NUMBER OF RELATIONS.

Let's get a rough idea of the potential number of interrelations in our imaginary system of **N** elements.

We name the first round bonds **Class-1 bonds**, the second round bonds **Class-2 bonds**, in general the **X**nd round bonds **Class-x bonds**, and the ultimate round bonds **Class-n bonds**.

It was said that the number of immediate first round bonds was: **N(N-1)/2**. In complicated systems where **N** is very big this formula can be simplified for calculations to **N²/2** as **N** will be much greater than 1.

Class-1 bonds

(binding two elements), elements contained = **2**; number of them will be = **N²/2**

Class-2 bonds

(binding two **Class-1 bonds**), elements contained = **4**; number of them will be = $(N^2/2)^2/2 = N^4/2^3$

Class-3 bonds

(binding two **Class-2 bonds**), elements contained = **8**; number of them will be = $(N^4/2^3)^2/2 = N^8/2^7$

.

.

Class-x bonds

(binding two **Class-[x-1] bonds**), elements contained = 2^x, number of them will be

$$= 2 (N/2)^{2^x}$$

.

.

Last **Class-n bonds**

(binding **Class-[n-1] bonds**); elements contained = N^n; number of them will be

$$= 2 (N/2)^{N^n}$$

These last ones will not bind to produce NEW different bonds for all contain the same components, but one can assume that they will fuse into **one** resonant bond of all these **Class-n bonds.**

The phenomenon of resonance along oscillators that vibrate with equal frequency is well known. One oscillator's impulses build the amplitude of the waves emitted by the other thus greatly increasing the intensity of them. Similarly it might be assumed that Class-n bonds will resonate enhancing the effect of each bond.

THE GRAND TOTAL OF NUMBER OF BONDS IN THE SYSTEM OF **N ELEMENTS** WILL BE:

$$\mathbf{N} = \sum_{X=1}^{X=\log_2 N} 2 \left(N/2 \right)^N \qquad \text{where } N = 2^x \qquad (1)$$

the number of bonds in the biosystem's castle of energies.

BONDS' CONTENT OF INFORMATION.

Information plays a paramount role in **control-energies.** Synthetic control will be used in the next Chapter IV to show this *dependence of control-energies on informational content.*

Assuming that information carried by the first bond of our model is one elemental bit (referring to bits of information as defined by the theory of information), the information carried by the bonds can be tabulated as follows:

Class-1 bond; number of elements $2 = 2^1$; bits of information = **1**

Class-2 bond; number of elements $4 = 2^2$; bits of information = **2**

Class-3 bond; number of elements $8 = 2^3$; bits of information = **3**

.

.

.

Class-x bond; number of elements $X = 2^x$; bits of information =x

.

.

.

Last bonds Class-n; number of elements $N = 2^n$; bits of information = **n**

The **n** bits of information in function of all **N elements** should be: **n = $\lg_2$ N.**

We can see that the *informational* content of the **total control-energy** of the system is that of one of the **last bonds** as it contains **only** the information of each **Class-n** *repeated*. Integration of **Class-n bonds** may intensify its *quantitative* power by no more than

$$2\,(N/2)^{N^n}$$

times that of one Class-n bond but will not add any bit of information to its *qualitative* capacity.

When **N** is sufficiently large the magnitude of these numbers defies imagination despite the fact that the initial content of information on the initial elements is the bottom line of **1.** Can you imagine the amount of information lodged in real systems whose initial elements may already contain a colossal amount of information? The physical expression of it could well be the expression of the intangible and undeniable realities emotions, intelligences and **wills** of living creatures.

INSTANTANEOUS FLOWS OF ENERGY.

As said the *energy flows* in the **castle of energies** of our imaginary system is practically *instantaneous* given the frenzied speeds of the elementary world.

The light speed of *energetic flow* is evident in biosystems. Man's processing of visual data has been estimated to be superior to 5,000 bits/sec. Memories including thoughts and emotions are examples fit to the occasion for experiences are recorded and stored in the genetic material as fast as they are originated. Reactions at the genetic level are of the order of one million to hundred million per second. Recently it has been reported an increase of the weight of the RNA proteins of the brain cells during the processes of learning and memorizing. Such marvels hardly conceived in ordinary dimensions are possible by the extraordinary speed of electronic activity, and apparently genetic speed adapts itself to it.

EMPIRICAL SUPPORT OF CONTROL-ENERGIES.

Universal evidence of control, *forced* as well as *inherent*, supports the existence of **control-energies**.

Control is an inexorable power of all systems that would be fatal should not elemental matter and energy be illuminated by the intelligence to make meaning out of information and to evolve intelligence to higher levels by association. The result of which is organization and harmony. In the acting and traveling of matter-energy, self-initiated association is beneficial as well as unavoidable resulting in subordination to and acceptance of the new more intelligent creations.

Harmony is ever more powerful in more intelligent systems and also more knowledgeable in the exercise of harmony. The universe has the greatest capability for it. No matter how extravagant organizations and systems develop within it, they cohabit in general harmony.

How ironic it would be that the most ignorant of systems or the non-intelligent *chance* be empowered with such inexorable control. The Creation, systems, organization and order, would succumb to blind forces of disharmony that we ascribe to evil. Not being the case, the Creation is simply good, brilliantly devised by its Creator in the simplest and most elegant of forms: *granting power to make meaning of information to the elemental matter and energy, and letting it free.*

57

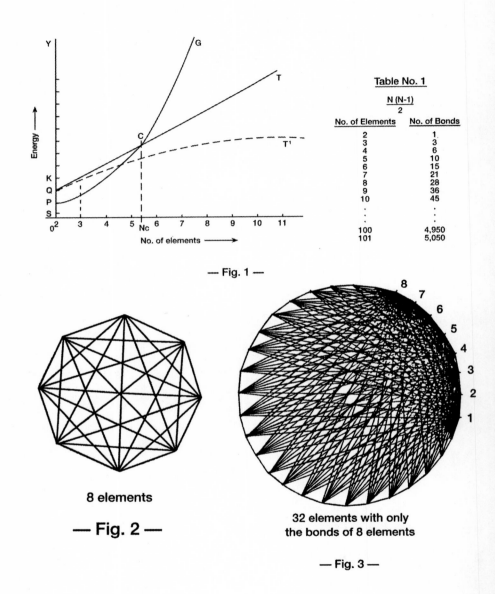

Table No. 1

$$\frac{N(N-1)}{2}$$

No. of Elements	No. of Bonds
2	1
3	3
4	6
5	10
6	15
7	21
8	28
9	36
10	45
.	.
.	.
100	4,950
101	5,050

— Fig. 1 —

8 elements

— Fig. 2 —

32 elements with only
the bonds of 8 elements

— Fig. 3 —

CHAPTER IV. - ENERGY AND INFORMATION.

The whole game of the universe is a dynamic interplay of energies controlling, subordinated or in equilibrium with other energies.

Until now I have purposely avoided defining *energy* because this thesis introduces new concepts that set the stage for an innovative revision of it. At this point let's venture to state that **energy is the capability to do work and/or to control other physical realities.**

This definition, while preserving the present notion of energy, encompasses the **control-energies** introduced by this thesis, the intrinsic control that a system exert over its components and the external forced control that organized energy exerts on less organized energy. These controls are everywhere. They are natural and spontaneous. Two specific aspects of the energy that cannot be justified solely in *quantitative*

59

considerations. It becomes unavoidable to accept that energy has *qualitative* features due to the *information* it carries. When this is accepted, automatically the *internal controls* within systems and their *external forced control* find a place and justification in the scheme of physical reality.

Before proceeding let us restate and expand some of the fundamental relations between *energy-control* and *information* already exposed.

The simplest natural bond has been explained using an imaginary bond **AB** of two *indivisible* elements **A** and **B**. Their *indivisibility* forces us to interpret the bond as a *temporal* joining or sharing of **A** and **B** during which the bond contains both elements. The bond's actions carry along the contained elements **A** and **B** and the bond's decision affects both **A** and **B**, while the decision and acting of one single element only affects itself and no others. The bond **AB** thus has a *control* superior to that of each separated element **A** and **B**. This control does not depend only in the *quantity* of energy but on the specific *type* of energy which is determined by its *content of information*.

Suppose now that **A** and **B** have the same quantity of energy. Take a bond of four elements identical to **A**: bond **AAAA**. Despite that it has double the energy than the bond **AB** it has no *inherent control* over **B** because **it** has none of **B**'s information and therefore cannot make *informed* decisions for **B**. Its power of decision over B is a *forced external control,* not an inherent control based in the meaning of **B**'s information. To have *inherent control* over **B** the bond should contain **B**. This *type of control* based in the *content of the information* of the energetic bond is a *qualitative* control rather than an amorph *quantitative* one.

Natural systems display **external control,** a power not intrinsic to any of the single elements or in the sum of them when they are independent of each other. It derives from the power of their interrelations. **External control-energy** is related to **information** because it results from the interrelations that are *informed energies* with more information than the elements have. The systems' **need** to extract energy from external sources arises when the *energy demanded by the interrelations* is superior to that which the elements can provide. **External control** appears when interrelations have been established and the organization materializes into a system. A tiny seed-crystal in a solution of its atoms obtains materials to grow from the solution because its integral **control energy** (its **will**) is more powerful than the energy of the particles on the solution that are not interrelated among themselves. Thus the seed-crystal forces them to join it in the formation of its lattices.

SYNTHETIC INTELLIGENCE, CONTROL AND INFORMATION.

Every tool man has invented is an ordered system to facilitate or to improve work. A more efficient use of the energy is accomplished by skillful mechanisms that create and coordinate extremely complicated *controls* needed to perform a task. The success of opening and closing a door lies in the right lock and key for it. Lock and key are an intelligent plan, a tool. The *energy* used to lock or unlock the door has no locksmith skills whatsoever, it has no information. The information *is* in the tool, the combination of lock and key.

Because there is an intelligent design at work, it is said that tools or machines are or have **synthetic or artificial intelligence.** Synthetic intelligence *elevates* the quality of energy to do a work that otherwise could not be done. At the same time it reduces the quantity of energy thereby needed for the job. Such effect is strikingly accentuated on *natural* intelligence for nature has evolved mechanisms far more clever than those produced by technology with a rather spectacular savings of energy.

Intelligence, according to this thesis, is *the capability to make meaning of information*. It is an inherent, essential character of physical reality. Synthetic intelligence is *not intelligence at all*

62

despite what its naming implies and the fervor with which some devotees attempt to prove that instruments, in time, will equate or surpass the natural intelligence of creatures. A few considerations will dispel whatever hopes in such chimera.

FIRST CONSIDERATION. (On origin).- The natural intelligence of physical reality spontaneously emerges without known external action, initially in elemental matter-energy and later in systems resulting from the interplay of its own social forces.

Synthetic intelligence does not spring on its own. The engineer's intelligence, a natural intelligence constructs it. The components or the whole of synthetic intelligence envisions no plan, skills or purpose. The engineer conceived, planned, drafted and put together the pieces of the tool foreseeing their functioning.

SECOND CONSIDERATION. (On operation). - The operation of synthetic intelligence is entrusted to external intelligent operators. The work of the cleverest computer depends on the programmer. When a foolish program is installed in the instrumentation or the computer it will produce a line of absurdities consistent with the *unintelligent* program so installed by the programmer. In addition the computer is unable to originate programs.

It copies them or derives them from others previously feed.

Instead natural intelligence works without external push. The intelligent routes that electrons run in their atomic orbitals, the cellular functions of living matter, the cosmic dance of galaxies are self propelled not in need of strange help that, on the other hand, is rather impossible to conceive as we saw in Chapter II. Moreover the *meanings* of such endeavors are incomprehensible to outsiders of the identity in question because natural intelligence is not *transferable* to another system.

THIRD CONSIDERATION. (On type of work). - A computer is not able to make judgments or to correct errors except when it has been already programmed to do so. Its works are purely mechanic: matching of patterns, and following instructions. *What patterns or instructions have been imposed on the workings of the universe?* The universe follows its own design and creativity as a whole and by each of its past, present and future constituents, elements and systems, every one *governing* itself and *harmonizing* with others. The second role of social harmony is probably more exacting than the first of self-government, and neither of them at the reach of a computer.

FOURTH CONSIDERATION. (<u>On control</u>). - *Control of operations* in synthetic intelligence has been *forcefully* implanted and specific *information* must be provided for its functioning. No part would operate by being glued, nailed, attached or linked onto the machine, and in the *proper way and spot*. All of that accomplished would be of no use without a supply of external informational control, for the machine would not work without receiving not only information but the *right information*. . . and intelligent commands. The notches of the key shall be the right ones to open the locked door; TV or radio emit pictures or sounds when synchronizing the proper waves; a telegraph transmits and records solely the pulses that had been activated. No information *given* amounts to no job. Actually the implanted *controls* are *not energy* and therefore, *no controls embodied in energy,* but rather, mere *information* lended by natural intelligence.

What a difference we see in natural energy! There is no glue, nails, or wires in any creature or inanimate thing controlling the *informed* make up or their operations. There is no wiring to external controls that will run or stop their doings. Nature controls well and alone its workings. Natural systems have their own internal controls and in addition, *select* and *control* the external energy and information they need. That has been the norm since the beginning of time and will no doubt continue forever. There is no synthetic intelligence with such amazing controls of itself and its external supplies.

FIFTH CONSIDERATION . (On supplied energy).- When unplugged, the computer stops. It is not energetically self-supporting nor is capable to plug itself into sources of energy or to fetch and control external energy. However great its *alleged* intelligence be (a most debated issue), the computer does not afford comparison with *real* **intelligence** and **power** of physical reality. The *alleged intelligence* of a computer has nothing to do with intelligence for it is simply mere *information, passive information.* On the other side nothing may halt the march of the Creation or the travelling of its elemental particles at light speed. The universe continuously expands claiming new spaces at speeds of the order of light-speed while simultaneously unfolding increasing number of novel orders, things and creatures. Its fertility is unending, incessant, ever increasing. Power, qualitative energy and information, emerge on it and from it as if *inexhaustible creation* was the very substance, essence and aim of its being.

SIXTH CONSIDERATION. (On meaning and purpose). - Another consideration is that of the stupidity of machines, computers included. These are faster than man; so are cars. They handle complexities that no team of men would be able to grasp, so do factories and manufacturing processes. They even err less than man, and in general what they are able to do nowadays is beyond any imaginable goal that man may set for himself. Nevertheless these admirable deeds are not understood by the computer but blindly performed. Their performance ought to be called at most *efficiency* but not *intelligence*. Nobody will argue that a hammer is more efficient than my thumb to hammer a nail. Computers are same in kind, instruments of man, as cars, radios, airplanes, missiles...and hammers. They are nothing more than an expression of man's power, a result of it and tightly subordinated to man's control.

SEVENTH CONSIDERATION. (On evolution). - Computers do not evolve, nor the essential qualities of *decision* and to *make meaning of information* will ever appear despite the most inspired innovations in technology. Time will run out of steam and machines will remain machines without any other evolvement than the *artificial* intelligence that man might lend them.

Reality, and evolution that emanates from it, are a design of Creation that man-made products cannot emulate for the simple reason that the *power of decision* and to *make meaning of information* are *intransferible, because they are essences of natural physical reality.*

Man possesses these in their highest degree despite his inability to transfer them to any apparatus, or for what it may serve to any other man. Precisely what Thermodynamics asserts: that man cannot create the perpetual mobile. While reality from the simplest forms of matter-energy in the Big Bang evolves in to many fronts, the greatest production man himself. Physical reality **is** the perpetual mobile.

Artificial things do not evolve. They corrode, break, disintegrate and render themselves useless, inactive or ineffective. Just the opposite that nature does evolving novelties and effectivities.

It is for this intransferibility of the essences of nature that *human concepts* cannot be considered to be physical realities. They are *information,* virtual images not more real than the images on a mirror to which cannot be attached any existence other than one in the mental world. To this category belong the concepts of *time* and *space* that don't pass the scrutiny of the above seven considerations. They do not *evolve* nor have the essential capabilities to *decide* or to *make meaning out of information*.

In short, any machine functions in borrowed intelligence, borrowed programs and borrowed energy. Nothing belongs to it. Its actions are not free but forced. They have no *power of decision* nor the faculty *to make meaning of information* as natural intelligence of physical reality has. This is **"the"** unbridgeable abysm that separates natural and synthetic or artificial intelligence.

THE EVALUATION OF SYNTHETIC INTELLIGENCE AND CONTROL.

Idle to say that to execute very complicated tasks machines or computers must gain in complexity. The reason is simple. A rich language of symbols is needed in order to carry out complicated programs to satisfy the intricacies of the job. Richer information in turn demands a greater number of communications and control mechanisms. Thus, the increase of synthetic intelligence inevitably brings out that of complexity of its mechanisms although not viceverse. A machine could be a most complicated devise of foolish mechanisms and useless parts.

Synthetic intelligence is evaluated by the **concrete information** that it is able to read out, process or produce. These activities certainly proceed under wired-in artificial controls. Synthetic intelligence **must** operate throughout controls, *it is embodied* in the controls and it is usually taken as synonymous to control. If synthetic intelligence is dependent on information and its assesment is that of information, then *synthetic control* shall also *be assessed in terms of information.*

There are methods to measure *information* in any type of structures and processes and thus synthetic intelligence is *measurable on the basis of the measure of such information* . By extension those methods are being applied to the evaluation of natural intelligence.

Let us set forth succinctly how this is done.

The **unit of information** is one **bit,** which indicates **one choice** between two possible alternatives: patterns, states, and items., etc, whatever the choices may be. Assuming two situations, one single **bit** is the information that by itself is enough to determine the situation chosen. For instance, a **light on** and **off** can describe two situations. If **light on** signals **danger** the absence of the light, **light off,** signals **no danger.** The light represents **one bit of information** because by being **on** or **off** it clearly indicates the situation at hand. It gives *unequivocal* information of the situation chosen when there are only two possible choices.

Digits **1** or **0** corresponding **1** to one situation and **0** to another are **one bit of information** because each symbolizes one of two situations.

Let us take a group of elements that can be arranged in *four* different patterns. **Two bits of information** suffice to specify each of the four patterns. With two lights, **two bits of information,** we are able to form four signals each symbolizing one of the patterns. Or naming **"light-off"= 0**, and **"light-on" =1**, the symbols for each pattern will be:

    00,   01,   10,   11.

Four patterns in total. Each group of two digits indicates the pattern chosen.

If the patterns or situations are *eight*, three lights, **three bits of information,** or three digits, are enough to make eight different signals, one for each pattern. The symbols will be:

000, 001, 010, 011, 100, 101, 110, and 111.

They represent eight patterns in total and there are eight different patterns themselves.

If the patterns are *sixteen*, four lights, **four bits of information,** or four digits are needed to convey sixteen different messages each representing a pattern. The symbols in this case will be:

0000	**0100**	**1000**	**1100**
0001	**0101**	**1001**	**1101**
0010	**0110**	**1010**	**1110**
0011	**0111**	**1011**	**1111.**

They represent sixteen patterns in total, and there are sixteen different patterns themselves.

And so on.

The reader may have observed that:

2 (2^1)	Situations required		1	**bit of information**	
4 (2^2)	"	"	2	**bits**	"
8 (2^3)	"	"	3	"	"
16 (2^4)	"	"	4	"	"

And in general

| n (2^x) | " | " | x | " | " |

The **bits of information** that represent all and each of n situations of a system are **x** the exponent of **2** that makes $2^x = n$. **One bit,** a unit of information, defines one of two situations $2^1=2$, 1 is the exponent of 2 that equals the number of situations to 2. The exponent cannot be a fraction. The next higher number of bits of information may represent the number of groups with one additional element.

NATURAL INTELLIGENCE AND INFORMATION.

We are familiar with statements such as : "this computer has several million or so many billion *bits of information*". As the same methodology has been applied to estimate natural intelligence we hear alike that a bacterium contains a few million *bits of information*, human genetic code 20 billion *bits of information* (2.10^9), or that the human brain has some 30 trillion *bits of information* (3.10^{13}). Intelligence of molecules, organs, systems or everything in physical reality is being assessed as *bits of information*.

When using the same method to measure synthetic intelligence and the intelligence of natural systems there is too much wrongly assumed and plenty missed. Natural situations, patterns or changes are items *essentially different* than the artificial ones, which are known and *predictable*. Natural ones are caused by free decisions. This fundamental error is due to not taking into account the *essences* of reality or how the *accidentals* relate to them. Natural systems have been stripped by present scientific views of their *natural* intelligence despite that its presence is stridently clear and profuse, indelibly impressed in the order and harmony of the Creation. The harmony of the universe and statistic laws tell us that the *individual* power of free decision although *unpredictable* -in general- is well used.

And, as natural intelligences are being measured with the same stick adopted for machines' intelligence, consequently with these egregious premises and approximations, man's intelligence sooner or later will lose the race against robots' on the basis of such measurements. A robot overstuffed with information is the **sole** requirement envisioned for its overpassing of human intellect and human control. **Never a greater absurdity!** at which we arrived not only by measuring synthetic and natural intelligence (if such is possible!) by the same process, but by disregarding the insurmountable barriers between *the natural* and *the artificial.*

The above method measures *artificial intelligence*, **that is** *information*. When such method is applied to natural systems the basic error is that it attempts to equate *the capability to make meaning out of information* with *information*. Such capability **is not information** but an *abstract quality* that extracts the **meaning** that the *measured information* has for the reality in question. This capability eludes instrumental measurement.

FREE POWER OF DECISION IS UNIVERSAL.

Opposed to instruments, natural realities are in command of their systems. They hold the strings of information, meaning and decision. This last factor carries a paramount weight, for under one particular set of circumstances the decisions of individual systems can still be diametrically opposed, and precisely *this* happens at every level of evolution. Elemental particles and natural systems are **individually unpredictable.** In contrast no engineer can install into a computer the capability to make *free unpredictable decisions.* Programs are pre-determined, circuitry wired-in, results mathematically linked to the data provided.

With the advances of technology there is an increasing consensus to view biosystems as **free** systems, their decisions arising from their innermost secret worlds and their interpretation of information made under absolute privacy and intransmissibility. This thesis states that the *principles* of action that apply to biosystems also apply to all physical reality; they are *fundamental principles* embodied on the entire universe. Matter-energy of biosystems is the same as that in the inanimate world and the difference of the freedom of their whole system is one of *quality-degree* rather than of *kind*. Snowflakes, none of which are alike, obviously *freely* decide how to grow their shapes.

Elemental particles and systems are unpredictable; their unpredictability is but a manifestation of the *freedom of their* **"integral control-energy"** reaching in man its highest expression, **free Will**, the anchor of social and moral responsibility. To postulate, as the quantum theory does, that *natural behavior* of elementary particles is **only** *statistically predictable* is the equivalent to admit : *that* **individual** *behavior...down to the photon* where history began, *is* **unpredictable**. The conclusion to be drawn from statistics is *that a majority on the set bends to certain trends, that nature is well behaved, systems following a general behavior* with *significant* exceptions. The **significant** *factor* is of paramount importance because it leaves standing the crucial facts: 1) that *unusual* behavior is **freely** exercised by *the few*, and 2) that *usual* behavior is **freely** exercised by *the most*. Both for the same reason: that they are made of the *same essences*. **One** dissenter in this statistical crowd suffices to hold the flag of **freedom of decision** of elementary matter...energy unavoidably *undefeated.* That is, the unpredictability and abnormal behavior of elementary matter...energy are declarations of the *freedom of decision* of all **natural** reality. *Predictability* is **general.** *Freedom of decision* is **universal,** is the *ultimate variable* of physical reality subordinated to none and nothing no matter how the issue is being aboard theoretically or empirically.

The innumerable things and creatures from the bottom to the top of the evolutionary ladder at a point in time are the most eloquent demonstration of freedom of decision. The exercise of **freedom to decide** and only **that** explains why identical matter (elementary matter-energy) is found un-associated in the interplanetary spaces while also being part of the human body as result of a faster track in the evolutionary path.

ASSESSMENT OF FREE DECISION.

Regardless the wrongs incurred on equating natural and synthetic intelligence when measuring both in terms of information, still the calculations to *estimate* natural intelligences on these basis are being widely used because they have proven to have a practical value. According to this theory they also have a theoretical validity and in addition they are a practical necessity for the following. No measurement method is feasible or units can be devised to assess *essences of reality* because essences are *abstract* and *not transferable*, two conditions that preclude physical measurement. They are known through their effects. Although *direct* measurement of natural intelligence and decision is not feasible, *indirect* assessment by assessing information, may be possible under the premises of this theory.

Previous chapters show that there is a correlation between the abstract and the concrete, the qualitative aspects of energy (decision and intelligence) and its content of information. Now, *information* opposed to the *essences* of reality is transferable, observable and measurable. It is the ponderable, the expressed, indeed the universal currency of concrete reality. If in fact there is a correlation between *information* and *intelligence*, in synthetic as well as in natural systems, then both can be assessed by the same method keeping in mind that the first is a *measurement*, the second a mere *estimate*. In addition, as **natural** **control** increases parallel to the increase of natural intelligence, natural control can be valued in relation to the same measurement of **information**.

Let's further clarify the concept of **freedom of decision**.

Freedom of decision could be tentatively defined -in *analogous terms* to those used in measuring information- as *the capability to accept or reject a situation or state, the decider being the sole controller of the decision*. Notice that control and freedom are inseparable concepts in natural events, the *controller* is *free to decide*. On the other hand *synthetic controls* have *no freedom* whatsoever. They are immediately subordinated to the supplied energy and information, and ultimately to a human operator that is the actual decider. Freedom of decision in synthetic intelligence is **nil** and therefore there is no subject to be measured. The *human operator* is the sole *free* factor when dealing with synthetic controls that are imposed or *forced* controls and not *free "control-energy"*. **No freedom** is to be expected **to appear** in the development of machinery either. The increase in complexity and improvements in synthetic controls do not render **freedom,** they render superior *forced controls* also these subordinated to man's control. Although machines in the future may yield amazing productions, these will still be the result of *non-free* mechanisms at each and every link in the chain of controls.

By the very constitution of *natural* systems any gain on **control** is a gain on **freedom of decision**. And because control is tightly linked to information, as it has been repetitively illustrated, *information* is too the basis upon which the *freedom of natural systems* could be evaluated.

A FREE UNIVERSE.

Back to the *initial* expression of freedom in the Creation. Elementary matter-energy might have the simplest **degree of freedom**. It could be to associate or not to associate with *compatible* energetic quanta or particles. Such universal faculty of *spontaneous selection* accounts for the unassociated matter-energy of the interstellar spaces when matter-energy is associated into cosmic systems.

Associations produce: 1) systems with higher *capacities and qualities* of *freedom* and 2) a greater number of *diverse identities* than the un-associated ones. Thus from N elements spring $N(N-1)/2$ binary bonds. And from these next round of bonds is greater in number and so on, more numerous at every round.

Therefore, by the process of association, **freedom** escalates on two fronts: 1) diversified systems having greater and more complex **freedoms,** and 2) **greater number of systems** at every new level of evolvement. We see this progression in the course of evolution. Few elementary particles produce the atoms of the periodic table. More than one hundred are recognized today. Plus *atomic freedoms* are greater than those of elementary particles. *Molecular freedoms* derived from associations of atoms are more powerful and diverse than the atomic ones; molecules are more numerous than the atoms that originate them. And so it happens to more complex molecules and structures evolving from those molecular blocks. It can be properly said that **evolution** is marked by **the increase of freedom in degree, diversity and proliferation.**

The evolvement of molecules culminates in the formation of nucleic acids and codes of life upon which living creatures develop. Here the expression of **freedom** is irrefutable. **Freedom** in creatures cannot be dismissed notwithstanding its *undetectability* by instrumentation. Creatures have *free Wills* dramatically expressed by their *unpredictable* actions.

Present Physics, every day with increased discomfort, interprets the concrete physical reality of the universe as a **non-free** item, systems put together by **chance** (by absolute absence of intelligence) including those systems in which *natural intelligence* and *freedom* is obvious. For if man is deemed to *be intelligent and free*, still all components of him are deemed **not** to possess natural intelligence nor power of decision. Their processes are supposed to be *wired-in* ones. The difference between a corpse and a living being attributed to a soul immune to scientific inquire. Souls are relegated the role of temporal guests of the universe. Medical remedies are ground on this interpretation of physiological processes. The medical advances to be expected with the right interpretation of physical reality are incalculable.

Upon the fundamental principles of Classic Physics, physical laws describe synthetic intelligences, synthetic controls and synthetic processes, in sum a *synthetic universe* rather than natural systems and events. Modern physics describe *the general* but is unable to deal with *the universal and the individual* at the most elementary stages of matter and action as well as the highly evolved systems. The crucial problem of science is the inability to interpret the *essence of reality* at its birth in the realm of our universe, in the form of elementary matter-energy. Take for instance the electron. A beam of electrons responds to *general statistical* predictions of the quantum theory but *individual* trajectories of a single electron are unpredictable. Science offers no reason, no justification for this *unpredictability*. It just misses the **essence** of the electron and **its fundamental principle of action**. And here it rests.

But by far the greatest obstacle to the current views of the universe is that it must explain at what point of evolution, and by what process, **freedom of decision** was produced, and it does not. Not a single evolutionary step is known that transforms **total lack of freedom** into **freedom of action,** and how it later evolves to culminate on a **free** man. Evolutionary leaps are fundamented on previous realities. Should *essential* qualities not exist then -in elementary matter-energy- together with their own rational evolutionary processes, as the one this thesis proposed, these *essential* qualities will not surface in the future. Freedom begets freedom, superior ones at every decision, as this writing describes.

Hence it ought to be concluded that the universe never has been a *non-free machinery* because at no place, nor time it underwent the transformation from a *non-free* to a *free universe* and a *biological world*. The seed of freedom of elementary matter-energy is but the beginning. **Freedoms** emerge everywhere at all times. Why might have God created freedom in the Paradise when He could -at once- have created it in a simpler form at the elementary level? And, in addition, why not give birth to a more rational Creation than the one spliced in incompatible sections of free and non-free creations as scientific views postulate? This theory contends that the lack of freedom of the inanimate world is only *apparent*, the result of harmonic social drives. Future calculated experiments eventually will confirm it.

This thesis reconciles contradictions by introducing the *whole* concrete reality, not solely its physical attributes, as subject of scientific study. It establishes and reasons that concrete reality has the *essential* capabilities to do *free decisions and make meaning out of information.* It sees the universe as a *free, intelligent* system and the biological world as a natural consequence rather than an unfit portion of it, a sort of sporadic miracle that includes humanity. Universal experience supports the proposals of this theory. This theory in fact is based on overwhelming empirical data offered by the Creation as we will see later in this book.

Our imaginary model is an attempt to reason:

1) the evolvement of power of decision and to make meaning out of information by the association of matter-energy, and

2) the evolvement of external control that systems exert to satisfy their energetic needs.

The quantized nature of matter-energy is being taken into account in the associating process.

Obviously this attempt to deal with reality and its creation cannot be other than an cursory rationalization to integrate the abstract and the concrete. We know well that interpretations of the abstract are merely guesses for practical application. For only its action is detectable, and no geometrical or mathematical model will reflect the intricacies of matter-energy in natural systems.

DIRECTION OF EVOLUTION AND FREEDOM.

Evolution runs towards more complex, intelligent and controlling systems endowed with greater freedoms when their social interactions settle in new orders and harmonies. We may ponder: Which of these factors: complexity, intelligence, control, freedom, order or harmony determines the direction of evolution? It is clear to this author that *freedom of decision* sets that direction, in fact **it is the power** that enacts and guides events to produce *realities* while harmonizing with others.

In the first place freedom of decision is not subordinated to any forces or faculties that would reroute action towards any particular direction. **Freedom** is the primal cause of action as well as the cause of its very **own** evolution and the evolution of natural intelligence. *No complexity, intelligence, or control can be produced without association;* no association without action and no action without *free decision* as discussed in our model. Order and harmony result from the coordination of social action that rests too on free decisions. Thus all arrows point back to the initial cause of evolution: *freedom of decision*. **The direction of evolution is determined by freedom of decision.**

Evolution itself **is** the perpetual work of **freedom** anewed and evolved in every created reality. Once a decision is made the future of evolution moves along its direction. Nothing can alter such decision or its consequences. Freedom of decision is a power of creation and successive decisions with their own intrinsic aims would not alter the initial direction or at least this author did not find any reason for such alteration. **Freedom** might be the **meaning** of the universe. Could it be the first *reality* to launch a free universe with uncontrollable power of creation?

The faculty of **freedom** is no less mysterious than **reality** itself. Therefore, it shall be accepted as we accepted the creation of concrete reality.

CHAPTER V. - DISCRIMINATORY ASSOCIATION OF ORIGINAL MATTER

This chapter will explore:

• how association in the elemental world might have occurred,

• under what drives or forces matter scattered everywhere was compelled to conglomerate,

• the reasons for the diversity of the resulting structures, and

• for its unequal distribution, certain areas being in a quasi absolute vacuum while matter fiercely competed in other areas for the same space.

What are the causes of this *discriminatory* distribution of the *same* initial cosmic materials?

It is obvious that whatever these causes were they and their input are of fundamental importance for the *association of matter* decided then, and still decide today, the shaping of the Universe, its operation, the evolvement of systems, the internal constitution of physical reality and the process of evolution. Revision of scientific *principles* is always a healthy practice and certainly an urgent one when questions accumulate unanswered by old adopted views. It seems now an appropriate time and place to address these questions with the new approach that this theory brings about **essential** factors of elemental matter and processes of cosmic evolution in both aspects, physical as well as abstract.

Today no logic mind would deny that man and living creatures -in their totality- are a *real* and *intrinsic* part of this Universe that originates and sustains them. Human intangible faculties, ideas, feelings, powers of creativity, wants and purposes lie properly within its confines and none beyond them. Man's *abstract concepts, emotions and morals* that find no place or provision in the current interpretation of physical reality are attributed to *his soul,* an entity out of the limits of scientific scrutiny. No explanations are found either for extensive biological phenomena, especially in the highest developed species defying the very foundations of physics. Their causes of action are attributed to *instinct* another word to substitute *ignorance* of those causes. Are those *uninvestigated faculties* actually an aspect of *universal reality*? *These issues* are addressed and rationalized by this *theory of systems* which postulates that elemental matter and energy are endowed with **power of decision, capability to make meaning out of information** and a **social drive** conductive to the evolvement of such faculties. **Freedom of decision** being **the ultimate variable** in the equation of physical reality.

Therefore, it is imperative to look for empirical support of such postulates. We will now attempt such a task with a simplistic and fresh overview of the *making* of the Universe and of its evolution by a *process of association* of matter and energy.

If some *essential* factors in the *processes of association* such as its *universality, intelligence* and *freedom,* have eluded us until now -judging by the monumental consequences they brought about- a new light on such processes should forever increase man's control of his own surroundings, of himself and the potential control he might have on the creation.

THE ORIGINAL UNIVERSE WAS FREE, INTELLIGENT AND SOCIAL.

Among several theories, it seems to be the prominent agreement that the universe came into existence 13.7 billion years ago in the Big Bang, a formidable explosion that happened everywhere *at once* and that gave birth to all matter and radiation of the cosmos.

Colossal forces at temperatures of about one billion degrees centigrade ejected matter in gaseous state throughout the spaces. What those forces were or where they came from has not been ascertained. The theory describes rather than explains the Big Bang not venturing back into the causes of it. Our Universe was thus born in a unique event of singular grandiosity and unconceivable dimensions, and from then its life started. *Life* indeed for the Universe is not immobile and permanent but ebullient with incessant activity and feverish creations. Was it at this original stage a *free, intelligent* and *selective* universe? It most certainly seems the case given the fact that it already showed *diversity, order* and *harmony.*

Matter then at such temperatures was wildly energetic but very simple in constitution. It could not have been otherwise. Everything necessarily would have disintegrated with the extreme heat. Thus, the Universe was mainly made of the simplest of components, ionized hydrogen (the nucleus of H with a single proton), electrons and elemental particles designed and confined to precise microspaces, their activity also mathematically framed in exacted intervals of time.

The explosion was of such a tremendous magnitude that the projection of matter to fantastic far-off distances produced a cooling effect across the immensity of the spaces. When this happened the gases *segregated* and *concentrated* into separate clouds of galaxies made up of smaller celestial formations of more concentrated matter. The Big Bang theory states that all galaxies were formed in a short time, in the opinion of some no longer than half an hour. That is not the typical picture of a cosmic catastrophe but rather the explosive birth of a spectacular *pattern of order and harmony* resulting from a universal, intelligent and *social* process. Such marvels that in addition occurred in an amazing short time *in the entire creation* cannot be attributed to the shuffling of **chance.** The probability of the formation of one single nucleus of hydrogen by chance is so slim as to require several times the life of the Universe to accomplish it, a span of time that would rather insure the destruction of any organization arising in a chaotic universe. But here we face a new born Universe entirely made up of *structured matter and energy* which furthermore has been organized into gigantic patterns of celestial bodies. The calculus of probabilities itself excludes *chance* in this astonishing scenery. Above all, action in this Universe seems to be guided by *freedom of selection* because the *same* type of elemental matter forming the galaxies also run *unassociated* in a practical vacuum between the cosmic aggregations.

There are about 10^{22} stars arranged, in number from 10^{11} (10 billion) to 10^{12} (one trillion), in galaxies. These galaxies in turn are congregated into fantastic clusters. Planets and other minor guests, satellites, comets and meteorites complete the part of the cosmos invisible to us due to their dim luminosity. Planets alone may exceed the number of stars assuming that our planetary system is fairly repeated along the rest of the creation.

As a result of the initial aggregations, the interstellar spaces, immensely larger than the celestial formations, were left with very rarified gas of an average density of 10^{-22} gr./cc, which is equivalent to the density of a *1 gr. of water vapor* filling a container of 10^{22} cc. This is approximately the volume of the Earth. Should we consider the dimensions of this isolation a *measure* of the power to refuse to associate?

The very opposite conditions dominated inside the stars. There, elemental particles and ionized hydrogen gathered in great concentrations attracted (we are told) by their *mutual gravitational forces*. As their distances shrunk, the attraction grew stronger and stronger to rampant violence, finally thrusting matter to fuse into highly compressed unions: the atomic nuclei. Particles in the nucleus remained bound by the most powerful energies known today: the strong forces. Under ordinary terrestrial conditions nuclear bonds are unbreakable. Should the conditions here be considered a measure of the power of association? According to this thesis the display of power *to associate* and *to remain isolated* combined is but a reflection of the power of *freedom of decision* in the elemental world.

Atomic nuclei are not mere conglomerates of matter and energy. Each one has a unique and very exquisite and accurate constitution with a range of characteristic energies. These are new patterns of organization and harmony of matter and action evolved with precision unmatched by any instrumentation ever conceived and despite unimaginable pressures. Gravitational forces, still unexplained by modern physics, lack the intelligence required to create the nuclei worlds of *selected particles* and *highly specific* energetic orbitals. Are gravitational forces simply an expression of the original elemental drive of matter to associate subordinated to an elemental power to freely decide whether to associate or not to associate?

Space and *time* shall be housed -so to speak- into the *abstract* faculties of organization of elemental matter and energy for the simple reason that they shall *precede* organization. Under this theory of systems, they are mere mathematical concepts, frames of reference, or virtual tools used by physical reality in their existence and evolution. Space and time, opposed to physical reality, are incapable of evolving into something else than what they are: *mental constructs, abstractions as a point, a line, a surface or a volume are.* What is indisputable is that such *mental constructs* are the same in all elemental matter when either isolated or in evolved systems. The atoms of the most remote stars have the same structures and timely actions as the terrestrial ones. Matter and energy seem to have identical *abstract concepts* of space and time all around the Universe.

Following the initial explosion, creation was instantaneously at work by a process of *association.* A *discriminatory or selective factor* was present here also for matter did not uniformly distribute itself out or within the celestial bodies of the galaxies. We may attribute this factor to *freedom.* In spite of this uneven distribution, matter and celestial formations kept a *social order* throughout the incommensurable spaces of the Universe familiarly labeled as regulated equilibrium. We may attribute it to *intelligence* for no other factor fosters order and equilibrium or social harmony on and among the micro and macroworlds of the Creation.

The dimensions and pattern of the Universe were not permanently set after the Big Bang. Originally the Universe was considerable smaller than it is now and from then the intergalactic spaces have been constantly expanding in all directions at rates comparable to the speed of light. It is not internally static either. Its components are mobile with velocities raging from that of light-speed down to every pace though possibly never reaching *rest*. As consequence of such traffic the Universe, so simple in its origin of elemental matter and energy, is becoming increasingly complex by further associations. It is evolving. It is alive. Periodically stars are born, maintain very active life and die. And so does every system and subsystem within its boundaries. The overall wondrous phenomenon is that novelty, evolution and complexity keeps ever producing new orders. The cosmos evolving direction, *the creation of order and organization* is always in irreversible progress. The Universe becomes more and more *ordered* because it unfolds novel orders at every detectable level from the infinitesimal to the astronomical.

Not until 15 billion years from the onset did the Milky Way make its appearance, the galaxy to which we belong and where the Sun shines among *one hundred billion* more stars. The Milky Way is spirally shaped with dimensions of 100,000 light-years long by 1,500 light-years tall. Our blue planet some 4.5 billion years old is swimming in a remote corner of that galaxy almost unnoticed in such a pompous Universe.

Let's get an idea of the extraordinary magnitude of such dimensions. Astronomical spaces are measured by light-years. Light travels at the speed limit of the Universe:186,000 miles/sec or 300,000 Km/sec. Nothing instrumentally detectable goes faster than light. Imagine your car running day and night for a whole year at the speed of light. At the end of the trip you would have covered **one light-year,** *about six trillion miles,* an insignificant **unit** in the vast context of stellar distances that are counted by *the hundred of millions of light-years.* (*Parsec* another commonly used unit is the length of the arc covered by the radius of the Earth in one sec/arc, which is equivalent to 3.26 light-years.).

Astrophysicists manage to express huge numbers in simple, accessible, elegant terms: the powers of 10. The radius of the *known* Universe, the greatest length ever estimated, is 10^{27} cm. This means a **one** followed by 27 zeros cm. In dealing with these mathematical symbols we should keep in mind that one single digit added to the exponent of 10 represents ten times the previous amount. Thus adding **one** to the exponent N of the Universe's volume 10^N will result in the volume of an universe **ten times** bigger than the present one. Adding **two** to the exponent will result in the volume of **hundred universes** equal to ours.

In our galaxy, the average distance between stars is 10^{19} cm. and they are estimated to be 10^{20} of them, about 10^{11} that is 100 billion. But the extraordinary astro-distances do not preclude stellar communication. There are galaxies *several billion light-years* far apart from Earth and these distant kingsfolks, that once were very much closer, are sending around continual messages in the form of electromagnetic radiation. Radiation inundates all spaces and because it travels at the speed of light we may consider it the swiftest message-carrier of the cosmos. The radiation of the Universe is a gigantic *social* enterprise!

Today we are recording messages mailed *five billion* years ago, long before the planet Earth came into existence. The Earth's age is approximately 4.5 billion years and we are receiving messages that remote galaxies mailed more than 5 billion years ago when Earth had not yet been born. Those peculiar messages convey, for one, the fantastic heavenly dimensions traveled by radiation; for another, facts and events that took place when our galaxy started to be shaped.

Who can deny that such stellar correspondence **is** a real communication among astros inclusion made with the *unborn* progeny? Cosmic mailing service has a permanency and reaching of communication commensurable with the grandeur of the Creation. A Creation bound by uncountable *social* drives! Those of the elemental matter-energy and those of the resulting systems. As we will see later.

CAUSES OF DIVERSITY AND ORDER IN THE UNIVERSE.

Accepting the origin of the Universe as stated by the Big Bang theory, let's ponder now the evident fact after its birth, that the Creation **is** *structured*. What and where are the causes of this peculiar *fashioning* of the universe that renders organization? Diversity and order should be preceded by discriminatory selective action, ordering control and a drive to associate. In other words, the *causes* of action must have *free decision, intelligence and social drive*. Where are such faculties of decision, intelligence and sociability enclaved if they are *not* part of physical reality as this thesis postulates?

It can be speculated that the mighty forces of birth-ejection causing *separateness* were *alien* to the Universe or we may consider that such forces were always *intrinsic* to physical reality. In either case when the explosion subsided, these forces had exhausted themselves in the task of the explosion remaining embodied in the matter-energy of the Universe. They had no place else where to go and no external forces ever after they had been claimed. Hence in the absence of any force alien to matter and pushing it to associate and harmonize within, we must concede that the *intrinsic social drives* of matter are the sole responsible for association, harmony and hence evolution and creation. Elemental matter and energy shall be accountable for its initial structuration and subsequent evolvement. The Big Bang theory does not offer other alternatives.

Energy and matter are not uniform, continuous substances as liquids appear to be in ordinary conditions. They are inexorably divided into precise amounts that do not admit further division. Energy in specific *elemental quanta*. *Matter is specific elemental particles*. They have a *granular* constitution. Any material or energetic quantity is *an exact number of elemental units*. There is no such thing as a photon and a half or fractional levels of energy. The atomic orbitals where electrons run are defined by precise levels of energy and it appears that when electrons jump from one to another they do it without traveling in what could be the intermediate levels of energy. They simply disappear in one level to appear suddenly in the other. Thus *identity of elemental matter* springs from this discontinuity as an essential aspect of *elemental physical reality.* One particle is itself and not another; energetic levels cannot be broken into fractions either. They are or they are not.

Let's come back to the interdistances and interrelations among the material and energetic units.

In addition to its *intrinsic discontinuity*, matter and energy are unevenly distributed in all spaces - as said- in the microworld, in the cosmic spaces and between those scales. From the almost matter-empty interstellar spaces constantly expanding, matter meets the other extreme in the core of the stars where temperatures eventually may arise 10^8 degree Kelvin. There, its concentration is such that the *solid state* got crushed losing the ordinary shapes and becoming like a plastic fluid heavily packed with *bare nuclei* and *blasting electrons* expelled from their orbits which are the frames that guarantee their atomic shapes. With matter-concentration goes annexed energy-concentration as one is but a transmutation of the other, two faces of the same coin.

Can it be said that gravitational forces were the initial *social* drive of matter? This Thesis supports that indeed they are actually *social* drives nonetheless a partial expression of more extensive and complex patterns of *social powers*, some imprinted in the original Universe and many and more varied ones unfolding in the evolving organizations.

The nature of gravitational fields of forces presents big questions still debated among physicists.

Newton envisioned gravitational forces as the strings that hold together the formidable architecture of the entire Universe. Of the 10^{22} stars, unknown number of

99

planets, satellites and scores of non-observable bodies, everyone enters the Newtonian theory. All are subjects of the Newton gravitational calculations together with every bit of dust and every particle integrating these microworlds. In describing those forces and giving them values, Newton was speaking about *universality*, moreover about *infinitude* and *eternity* following the religious tenor of his times. The Big Bang theory came much later. Gravitational forces, according to his view, operate *at distance* throughout the *space* which he considered to be an *immovable reality* occupied by an hypothetical fluid - *ether*- whose existence has never been proven.

He arrived to his famous formula in 1577 by extremely simple mechanical considerations. It reads: $F = M \times M'/k \times d^2$ where F stands for the gravitational force among two bodies of masses M and M' whose distance is d, K being a constant depending on the medium. The formula is valid in ordinary dimensions and still widely used in astronomical calculations. Newton penetrated with incredible approximation the value of gravitational forces that worked out the admirable regulations of the cosmic formations and the rest of the Universe. A touch of grace that placed him in close contact with the universality and essences of reality. Invisible, near and remote, future or past, those forces of matter were tremendous realities in Newton's mind and his discovery was a gigantic feat upon which progress had been made possible.

The concept of space and gravitational forces have been modified by the Einstein theories. For Einstein the *space* is a continuous *reality* that can be distorted by the fields of forces created by *masses*. In his view gravitational force does not operate *at distance* but its *apparent* effect on material bodies is nothing other than the effect of inertial forces. Material bodies are impelled to move on the *distorted spaces* pulled by their own inertia. Thus Einstein adjudicated to *space a real existence* and endorsed it with properties, variability and relations to other *physical realities*.

Under either view gravitational forces can be termed *social forces* provided that we interpret them as being originated by *physical reality*. Social order in the controlled microworlds and in the astronomic dancing shall result from intelligent action aimed to preserve individual existence and collective co-existence. Gravitational forces per se or distorted spaces fall short of fulfilling such demands. There is too much intelligence displayed in the *order* and *diversity* of the initial violent Universe and much more lately in progressive levels of cosmic evolution. The only avenue to *order* is the existence of an *intelligent social* drive intrinsic to elemental matter and evolving throughout a *consistent process* of association. Yet *diversity* calls for a power *universally* distributed although *unevenly* exercised, and that is a *social drive* subordinated to the *freedom of decision* of elemental matter.

HOW THE WORLD OF THE SMALLEST EVOLVED.

Initial matter consisted mainly of photons (units of light), electrons (units of negative charge with almost nil mass) and protons (nuclei of hydrogen of mass=1 charged positively). We enter now in the world of the smallest and measurements are expressed by the powers of 10 with negative exponents. Thus 10^{-24} gr. equivalent to $1/10^{24}$ gr. is the weight of an electron, $0.53.10^{-8}$ cm. equivalent to $0.53/10^8$ cm is the radius of the orbit of the electron. Angstrom a unit used to measure wavelengths of radiation has a value of 10^{-8} cm.

Orders and organizations evolved in the microworld by *association*, every creature having an active role in the play. Association of elemental particles gave origin to the underlying micro-structures of matter, the atoms, and also called elements. About one hundred elements are all that the Creation could produce. From these fundamental building blocks everything else was formed.

An atom consists of an extremely dense central nucleus *almost indestructible* where practically all its mass reside and electrons circulate in orbits of diameters about 10,000 times larger. Electronic orbits are actually energetic states defined by their distances to the nucleus. Although electrons and protons attract each other, electrons do not precipitate into the nucleus. Centrifugal ones, due to the fantastic velocities at which they run their trajectories, compensate these forces. They circulate *several thousand billion times* around the nucleus **every second.** You can imagine the electronic turmoil that is going on in our bodies; and for what matters, going on in the whole Universe. Because the mass of electrons is irrelevant and they are so far from the nucleus, the atom is almost empty space.

Nuclei are made up of protons and neutrons (elemental particles similar to the proton without electrical charge). The number of electrons and protons are equal. Thus, the whole system is electrically neutral. Atoms have an identification number, so to speak, the Atomic Number, that indicates the number of protons lodged in the nucleus and therefore the number of electrons in their orbits. Atoms each one having a proton more than the previous one are arranged in the Periodic Table of Elements. Those with Atomic Number close or superior to 100 are unstable and most of them artificially obtained. Due to this constitution we can see that the main problem in the creation of atoms is the creation of their tightly bound nuclei. Let us see how this is done.

Maria L. Costell Gaydos

HYDROGEN, the lightest and simplest of the elements was the first atom in the Universe. Presently it is still the most abundant, almost 75% of the total weight of the creation. From it other elements originated by nuclear reactions in the stars and this production of atoms continues through the ages along the entire universe and by the same processes. Those that yielded the original atoms after the Big Bang are repeated in the stars at all times. What happens in the stars now and then is unequivocally revealed in the radiant stellar energy emitted by their nuclear reactions.

The stars are, in the variegate array of celestial formations, the only spot apt for the manufacturing of atomic nuclei that met the conditions of such undertaking. Elemental particles and hydrogen in order to create heavier nuclei ought to be compressed into densities 10^{12} times that of water, which can be compared with the densities that might develop if one million tons of metal were squeezed into one single cc. The interrelations, collisions and reactions resulting in this unimaginable pressure would rise the temperature needed for the singular cooking out of which protons and neutrons will consolidate forever into atomic nuclei. Atomic nuclei are assembled there at temperatures of ten million degrees centigrade raising to one billion, and pressures of approximately 150 million lb./sq.in.

There is no *material* tool that could crush *matter* to those extremes without collapsing itself. Under such pressures the very structure of matter, the edifice of electronic orbitals that secure the atomic shapes, would shatter like a crystal tower by bombing. No device would resist such atrocious temperatures or would contain the escape of matter invigorated by such tremendous energies. However gravitational forces handle the task with ease by developing the adequate controls within the stars that thus become the proper pressure cookers of the cosmic materials.

Gravitational forces are irrepressible. Action might have begun by a tenuous attraction among particles and atoms. The closer they came, the stronger they were thrust together. Newton's formula teaches that their attraction increases inversely to the square of the distance. With nothing to stop them, they would accelerate and amass in stellar quantities, the violence of their embraces would eject electrons out of their orbitals, assuming that the lovers are still hydrogen atoms. Spaces among particles would be reduced to zero; material structures would be crushed to a heavy plastic gas of compact nuclei where no form is possible since no rigidity stands those rigors. Meanwhile electrons running vertiginously would act as projectiles on the nuclei, which inexorably would be struck on account of their compactness. Their positive charges which attract electrons further adding to the impact. Then the nuclear reactions start and they release a considerable amount of energy that continuously increase the temperature of the set up.

Gravitational energies can control the otherwise explosive energies produced, superior to any nuclear weapon ever conceived. That gives the star some sort of frontiers to initiate and protect its internal organization. Now, new *social forces* enter the scene, the *strong nuclear forces* that for some reason spring when distances among protons and neutrons are of the order of 10^{-23} cm. Strong forces among two protons are 10^{39} times their gravitational ones. (Here I am speaking of two single protons to illustrate the relation. In considerable amounts of matter the effect is not the same as among two singular protons. Because of the strong forces, protons and neutrons are glue forever in the nucleus even at the ultimate event of the disintegration of the star. The strong forces therefore seal permanently the marriages on the atomic nuclei. To bind very massive nuclei are needed more powerful gravitational forces and these are generated when the accumulation of matter is enormous. Thus the mass of the star has a direct impact on the type of nuclei created.

The nucleus as far as Chemistry is concerned, is completely inactive. Its components are firmly bound together by the strong forces greatly superior to those holding the electrons in the orbitals. These are maintained by the electrical fields between the nucleus and the electrons. Chemical properties depend entirely on the *social* activity of the electrons. Their number and their energies determine the chemical *links* with which are intertwined the molecular fabrics. Atoms communicate among themshelves through their electrons and by their *associations* generate the molecules. The next Chapter deals with these new levels of the *social* play.

Chemists -as said- have included all existing atoms in the Periodic Table of Elements. Each atom occupies a square in the Table and it is designated by an **Atomic Number** that has a significance greater than merely indicating the square number. It describes the total structure and chemical properties of the atom in question. The Atomic Number is the exact number of electrons in the atom and the number of protons in the nucleus. Neutrons may vary given place to different so called isotopes. These have different mass but still have the same Atomic Number and the same atomic properties. To simplify formulations atoms are named by symbols of one or two characters that are abbreviations derived mostly from their Latin names.

The world of atomic elements is created in its entirety out of **Hydrogen** throughout nuclear **associations.**

Hydrogen, symbol **H,** whose **Atomic Number** is **1,** has one proton and one electron. Deuterium and tritium are two isotopes with one and two neutrons incorporated to the nucleus respectively. Energy or collision may eject the electron out of the normal atom of Hydrogen leaving the nucleus isolated with a positive charge, which is actually the *proton*.

Helium, symbol **He,** of **Atomic Number 2,** contains two protons in the nucleus and two electrons in orbit. That is its nucleus is the sum of two Hydrogen nuclei. Most of the stars including the Sun are mainly a mixture of Hydrogen and Helium, the easiest nucleus to obtain. The constant nuclear reactions from these two elements yields energy in the form of heat and light that gives the stars their typical luminosity.

Once the nucleus of Helium is obtained in the star, a chain of reactions is possible by collisions with it. The association of three Heliums give birth to Carbon, symbol **C,** of **Atomic Number 6,** an atom of transcendental importance on Earth, for it is the axis of organic life. The predominant ingredient of every organic molecule is Carbon. Organic Chemistry has become in the last century the Chemistry of Carbon.

Next, nuclear compounding of Carbon with another Helium originates Oxygen, symbol **O,** of **Atomic Number 8.** Then by reacting Oxygen nuclei with Helium the resulting product is the Neon nucleus. Symbol of Neon is **Ne**. **Atomic Number 10.**

With Neon and another Helium a new element results, the Magnesium, symbol **Mg**, of **Atomic Number 12**. And so on. Succeeding additions of nuclear protons to each element produce the subsequent elements of the Periodic Table. Complicated structures are born from simpler ones.

Collisions analogous to the above mentioned generate the first 26 elements of the Periodic Table. Iron, symbol **Fe** has the **Atomic Number 26**. There after it is necessary to hit the preceding atomic nuclei with *high speed neutrons* in order to create more complex nuclei. At this point *neutrons* have been generously generated and energized in the previous reactions that gave birth to the 26 elements. And with the new weaponry available and ready for action the production of the remaining atoms of the creation does not pose any problem. Simply a new *social* game of matter with a denser membership.

The following are a sequel of a few nuclear reactions. The up indices stand for the combined number of protons and neutrons in the nucleus. The **Atomic Number** is indicated down

$$H_1^1 + H_1^1 \rightarrow He_2^4 + \text{Energy}$$

$$He_2^4 + He_2^4 + He_2^4 \rightarrow C_6^{12} + \text{Energy}$$

$$C_6^{12} + He_2^4 \rightarrow O_8^{16} + \text{Energy}$$

$$O_8^{16} + He_2^4 \rightarrow Ne_{10}^{20} + \text{Energy}$$

$$Ne_{10}^{20} + He_2^4 \rightarrow Mg_{12}^{24} + Energy...\text{and}$$

so on.

All elements of the creation, with no exception, are those listed in the Periodic Table. That is so because protons and electrons are **units** that cannot be fragmented therefore intermediate elements with a fractional Atomic Number do not exist. The Periodic Table actually includes about 105 elements although the latest ones and some added posteriorly have been obtained artificially and have a very short life. Very complex elements are unstable. Possibly more elements will be made in the future with particle accelerators (cyclotron, bevatron, are the names of these sophisticated instruments) but having less stability and consequently less usefulness, presumably this line of research will not go too far.

The reader may find difficulty accepting the conclusion that only 105 atoms are all that the universe can offer. Is it not possible, you may ask, that in some distant galaxy one lucky star gave birth to an unfamiliar set of elements? As far as we know, there is no such possibility. The nucleus structures are very stable and practically indestructible excepting for a few radioactive materials. They are bound by the *strong forces,* the greatest forces in the universe. Nuclei retain their constitution even in the extraordinary events of SUPERNOVA explosions and when undergoing chemical reactions of the *nuclear* type.

In all property, atoms are the indivisible blocks of all matter.

But besides their own internal constitution, the atoms speak for themselves, from every corner of the Universe and from many eras since the Creation throughout stars' radiation that travel to Earth and whose trips were initiated one, two, several billions of years before their arrival. Atoms' messages are received and translated in the *spectroscope* whose fundament is very simple. When light passes across a triangular prism, as the figure 1 shows (at the end of this Chapter), it splits into a spectrum of colors each having a different wavelength, an occurrence caused by the fact that the prism bends the light more or less proportionately to its wavelength. Basically the spectroscope is a light analyzer.

All matter absorbs and radiates energy and that energy transports information. When energy is given to a metal it becomes heat. It is the captured energy that raises the temperature. The metal gives away energy while cooling. And the interesting phenomena is that the energy absorbed or radiated is characteristic of the *specific* material and exacts its atomic organization. Those radiations accurately describe the whole atomic edifice.

A container cannot take or give more liquid than that of its own capacity. The analogy applies to the case of energy. Electrons in the atoms are disciplined to rotate in orbits (energetic states). They do not wander around, but they can be excited to jump to larger orbits by accepting or borrowing energy. Later they may return to their normal paths and they release *just* the same amount and type of energy they took to perform the jump. In both events the energy absorbed or emitted defines the difference of energy between both states. As no two electrons have the same energetic state the spectrum is a display of the electronic orbitals, the internal atomic organization.

We may plan the spectroscopic analysis in two ways: leading to a *spectrum of emission* or to an *spectrum of absorption.* The first by directly analyzing the light emitted by an excited material, for instance, heated metal. The second by interposing the substance to be analyzed in the path of a source of *known* light and *known* spectrum. The light will be deprived of certain radiations, which will appear in the *known* spectrum as dark lines. This spectrum is the exact negative of the first.

The series of lines projected into either spectrum is characteristic of each element of the Periodic Table. Each atomic edifice differs from all others and so the pattern of lines can be very complex for elements of high Atomic Numbers. The pattern is *highly specific;* no imitation is possible by any other atom or any combination of substances. **Each** spectrum is **one** structure. It amounts to a signature that does not admit forgery, a unique fingerprint.

Trace of products as small as 1 billionth of a gram are detected by spectrographs, in any molecular form, state, distance, or place they may be, for atoms always emit their own characteristic radiations. Nor does Carbon on Earth differs from Carbon seated in the limit of the Cosmos. Today the atomic structures of all elements have been described, measured, weighted to infinitesimal approximation. Conclusively, at this level of association there are no more atomic systems than those encased on the Periodic Table.

THE ASSOCIATION DRIVE IS INTRINSIC TO PHYSICAL REALITY.

Radiation of the Cosmos eloquently tells what happened after the Big Bang: the creation of patterns of organization in the entire micro and macroworlds. Subatomic particles associated into atoms **selectively** choosing their mates and number of possible associations, not only rendering **spatial orders** but also **ordered activity**. Matter and energy of the Universe simultaneously arranged itself in harmonic equilibrium, from isolated elemental particles to conglomerates of stellar formations whose immensity defies imagination.

113

The creation of social order implies:

- **intelligent selectivity** by each and every element of such order to estimate choices,
- **conception of space and time** -*common to all reality*- to design patterns of organization and timely activity.

Blind energy and the empty notion of **chance** do not breed but chaos. And the just born Universe, inundated by radiation of precise wavelengths, exquisite conceived matter, and grandiose astro bodies, was the antithesis of chaos. This was simply the beginning, the lower level of organization upon which uncountable and unimaginable ones evolved.

The theory of systems postulates that the order and harmony of the Universe has its roots in elemental matter and energy that has an **essential social drive** manifested in the associations it creates. Isolated elemental particles reinforce the fundamental principle of the theory: that the faculties of matter and energy are subordinated to the *freedom of being used or not being used.* On this ultimate **freedom of decision** rests the *diversity* of the Creation.

CONCLUSION: SOCIAL DRIVE OF PHYSICAL REALITY IS RESPONSIBLE FOR ASSOCIATION, HARMONY AND CREATION.

Subatomic particles associated into atoms SELECTIVELY, choosing their mates, the number of them, the patterns of grouping and the number of possible associations, not only rendering a spatial order but also orderly activity. Although electrons and protons attract each other, electrons do not precipitate into the nucleus because of their trajectories at fantastic velocities. They circulate *several thousand billion times* around the nucleus EVERY SECOND. Can you imagine the electronic dancing that is ongoing in our bodies? And what about that of the whole universe?

The picture of the Cosmos eloquently tells what happened after the Big Bang: the creation of ORDERLY patterns and the creation of social ORDERED activity throughout SELECTIVITY AT EVERY LEVEL of matter and energy and along every inch of the creation.

What and where are the forces of ORDERING and SELECTIVITY?

In the absence of any magical force alien to matter and pushing it to associate and harmonize, we must concede that the intrinsic drives of matter are responsible for ASSOCIATION, HARMONY and thence CREATION.

115

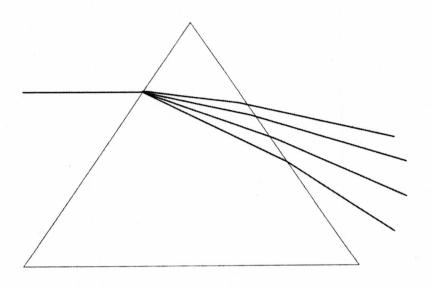

Figure #1

CHAPTER VI. - GENERAL AND UNIVERSAL LAWS.

Let's now dwell on the notions of disorder and order. The first is connected with *unpredictability*. Not one section of a disorderly area or set up can give indication of the happenings in some other section of that area. There is no logic or method that can be followed in disorder to make predictions. Instead *order* is repetitive, regulated, predictable. We can guess in an *orderly* series of numbers the value of any one by applying the pre-established rules of the succession. In consecutive *even* numbers the occupant of place 10 is certainly the number 20 and always will be. Numbers are subjected to *universal* rules consistent with the terms that define their orders. These are *universal laws* because they do not allow for exceptions. Laws that describe natural phenomena or activity have room for exceptions and are called *general laws*.

117

Classical theories of Physics teach us that immutable and universal laws regulate nature. Pure water boils at 100^0 C; therefore, pure water from any source, under equal experimental conditions, will repeat the trick of boiling at the same temperature. It is said to be preordained in the water's molecular constitution. A particular cause invariably produces the same effect. The Classical Universe is logical, inflexible, *deterministic*. Modern Physics depart from this position. For instance the Quantum Theory deals with *general*, probabilistic, statistical laws, basically establishing that there is a fundamental *uncertainty* in the description of the individual elemental particles. Such uncertainty will not break with more accurate instrumentation for it is intrinsic to the nature of physical reality. Determinism is loosing ground with the new directions of thought. But in sharp contrast with this stance an amazing number of scientists concur with the *philosophical* view that every bit of the Universe operates under *the same* laws and forces. Hence, scientific plans are geared to discover those laws and energies and to formulate a final grand unified theory that will explain *all* phenomena.

I said *philosophical,* and ironically so, because the scientific approach is *empirical* in thought and method, and Empiricism is a philosophical doctrine conflicting with those aims to discover the *universal*. The empiric method consists of compiling specific facts that are extrapolated into a general law that ultimately must be sanctioned by calculated experiment. Don't be mislead! Factual reports lead no further than to statistic conclusions far from *universal principles*. Empirical data assumes that physical reality is only *that* which is instrumentally detectable and this premise precisely ignores, eliminates and rejects *the universal,* the *essences* of nature and therefore the possible ground of *universal* laws.

The search for the *universal* is a different philosophical enterprise altogether. That is clear for the scientist that now shall change method by using *thought experiments* helped by *mathematical and geometrical auxiliaries*, both *abstract* tools, to interpret squarely *concrete* physical reality. No abstract aspect of Nature enters the equation. The *universality* of these mathematical and geometrical tools is based on *definition* and not *on Nature.* Thus a virtual scheme of reality created by the scientist is superimposed in the description of nature. In these serious inconsistencies of principle lie the main problems of Physics. Einstein had good reason to state "a scientist is a poor philosopher." With this sort of justification for the deficiencies that can be encountered in these writings, let's now summarize our philosophical position about the *laws of Nature* and its consistency with the postulates of this theory.

This theory does not agree with the above total or partial *deterministic* views of science that considers matter and energy to be under the mandates of natural laws. *It retains instead that laws do not exist.* There are no *independent laws* to which physical reality is subordinated. The so-called *laws* are exclusively *descriptions* of the activity of matter-energy. It cannot be otherwise because all action depends on the *free decisions* of elemental matter-energy or systems evolved from it. Free decisions are unpredictable. All that can be said of the laws of natural phenomena is that they are *probabilistic* and *general.* The term *universal* is reserved for the *essential* features of elemental matter and energy which are also present in the systems that evolve from it. The rationale behind it is this: The innovative orders of evolution, the evolvements of new qualities of matter-energy shall contain the *universal essences* of it. This was explained in Chapter II with an imaginary model, a bond AB between two elemental components A and B. The bond AB must necessarily inherit from its components A and B the *essential* capacity to make *free decisions* and *meaning out of information* because is made up of the *same energy* of A and B. In addition, because the process of association *increases the content and quality of information* such capacities evolve to higher levels of complexity and power. The bond AB is more free and more intelligent than the original two elements A and B. The *social drive essential* to the elemental components A and B shall also be inherited by the bond AB and evolves to higher levels of sophistication for the same reason. Thus, the social drive preserves its *universality,* as well as, the capacity to make *free decisions* and *meaning out of information.*

This sketched conceptual model gets flesh and body in physical reality where *essences* of reality are *immanent* and *universal*. They are universall*y manifested in concrete events,* as it will be repetitively observed and analyzed in examples upon examples in the following chapters. Such manifestation from elemental matter to man, proves the tenets of this theory. Science has missed the crucial *universal* aspects of Nature by purposely and systematically dismissing *the abstract, which naturally* escapes instrumental detection. Consequently science dismisses the link between the abstract cause, *the identity*, and the effects resulting from it.

Previously we discussed the *universal manifestation* of the *essences* of elemental matter and energy. Now we will venture in the present Universe, a Universe integrated by *systems* and we will focus on the manifestation of the *universal essences of systems*. Thus, in this new phase this theory will expand its postulates about *elemental* matter and energy into the *universal* description of *all* physical reality.

THE SELECTIVITY OF THE UNIVERSE.

Chapter III explored the *order* in the initial Creation and *that* order excludes *chance* and *blind forces* exterior to elemental matter-energy as the cause of association. Any association whose end product is *social order* requires *processes* with a sort of intelligence not possessed by *chance* or blindness. Moreover, an *order* so extent as that of all elemental matter of the Universe. We saw that the cause of association is intrinsic to elemental physical reality not extrinsic to it. The *association* of matter must be preceded by *essential social* drives, which display a definitive *selective* action conductive to *order*. Selectivity is a complex affair. There are various implicit aspects in the selective action of elemental matter and energy.

FIRST. - To associate. - That in itself *is* a selection. Whereas it has been proven that all elemental matter is the same and therefore all capable of association, the lack of association of part of it suggests that matter selects not only the partners with whom to associate but also the actual *act* of association.

When elemental particles associate, association has been preferred to the alternative of wandering around in randomness. The state of isolation allows the particles an unlimited freedom of movement, while association cuts individual activity to the limitations of one particular order or pattern. This *apparent reduction* of freedom seems to contradict the fundamental premise of this theory that proclaims that freedom is inviolable. We will elaborate on this matter later and prove the opposite: association results in an increase of freedom. What are the reasons to associate? Are these reasons or logic based on information, processing of information or some *intuitive* powers of nature located on an *abstract* level? Do the particles know that the resulting system will have more freedom than the individual particles have? Whatever the answers <u>elemental matter has the power to associate</u>.

SECOND. -<u>Selection of the associates</u>. - Constituents of the association are not picked up at random but under severe scrutiny. For instance let's consider the associations of the microworld. The initial Universe materialized very few *patterns of order:* only the 105 atomic nuclei listed on the Periodic Table, which cannot be stretched further because more complex elements are unstable. The matter of the *entire* Universe, in frenzy activity at light speed, for 20 billion years, had exhausted its patterns of *association* in solely 105 atomic designs. That is all that it could produce. This figure does not excite the imagination but surely tells a transcendental fact, the *precise selectivity* with which elemental matter associates. Whatever powers activate such selection, they are the same for *all* elemental matter and energy of the Creation irrelevant of space and time. From the remotest regions of distant galaxies to the closest of planets no other elements besides those 105 are found. All elemental matter selects its associates.

THIRD. - <u>Selection of interrelations that hold the association</u>. - Interrelations in the association should satisfy the many requirements imposed by the participants in both dimension, the concrete and the abstract. The task to negotiate suitable accords among members becomes more difficult when the number of them increases and thus grows the complications of the set up. Nevertheless, bonds in atomic nuclei are not confused. Strong forces binding protons and neutrons in the nuclei of diverse elements are *characteristic* of each one of them, and exactly the same in the nuclei of the original Universe as in the nuclei of today. Radiation from far away times and spaces tells the story unequivocally.

Notice that in the interrelations we are facing the *creation* of novel energies, *the bonds*. Which is to say that such *creative power* is *selective*. This brings us to the fourth and most mysterious aspect of *selective* sociability: the selection of future superior orders, structures and systems, which are certainly not embodied in the components. These are mere pieces of the total puzzle. Nevertheless, previous elemental matter has selected its interrelations in the association.

FOURTH. - <u>Selection of the final structure to be produced</u>. - Our model of the development of a system shows that the number of interrelations among components increases geometrically with the number of components involved in the bonds. In the final structure there is an unprecedented number of *selected* relations with the purpose to secure harmony among associates, bonding energies, the whole with them and they with the whole. These relations arise from free decisions. If the *selective* interrelations *among* the components in the association, *at once,* were not mysterious enough, what can we say of the *selective* net of interrelations that should *anticipate* the final organization to be produced? Did initial elements and each of the successive bonds foresee the final pattern and fashion their *free* relations accordingly? Has elemental matter a *purpose*? It seems so, given the organization in all phases of cosmic evolution.

Finally, we may consider this, to speak about *selectivity* is to speak about *identities*.

The Universe could have erased the above four steps of selection by erasing *identities* altogether. Selectivity would not be needed if *individualities* did not exist. *Elemental* matter and energy must have been endowed with *identities* since its origin when *selection* is here, and

125

well, and there is no explanation for its appearance if not by a rational process of inheritance from elemental matter. Assuming the existence of *elemental identities*, association of individual identities without power of selection would make no sense; a show without audience; information without processors of it. This Universe is a clever one that *does make sense* and does not contradict itself. And so *identities* and *selectivity* come one with the other, sine qua non, hand in hand as *universal* features of *elemental* physical reality and action. *Identity*, a universal abstraction. *Selectivity,* the expression of its will, intelligence and social drive.

EVOLUTION AND SYSTEMS.

This chapter is an inquiry on systems which is equivalent to an inquiry on evolution.

The *faculty to associate* does not vanish by the fact of association. We see it evolving and in continual operation. After an order has been perfected, another order appears. Order in the Universe is not a one shot process but a continuous orderly association of its unresting components. Evolution is the unfolding arrangements of matter and energy into new orders, organizations and structures, which bring with them new qualities and *new identities*. Experience tells us that evolution or natural association never stops, that is, *sociability* is a *permanent* quality of physical reality, in elemental matter and in the systems derived from it.

Most physical reality appears in the form of systems. The Universe, a system in itself, and every subsystem within it are in continuous evolution, elements and systems harmonizing among themselves. Relying on evolutionary data I expect to interpret the nature of systems and validate the previous interpretation of *elemental* matter-energy, that is, the principles of this theory.

Luckily for this work, the evolutionary rate is not the same along the Universe and that variety of evolutionary phases gives away the details of the systems' evolvement. For example, at this very moment, photons and other subatomic particles wander in the interstellar spaces not yet near association, and atomic nuclei of the entire Periodic Table are being created on big and small stars just as it happened shortly after the Big Bang.

The evolutionary disparity is even more colorful on Earth where inanimate matter coexists with animate creatures. Two distant stages of evolution side by side. The first arrested since the birth of the planet in contrast with the progressive vitality of the second. Land and seas are populated with millions of plants and animal species belonging to each spark of life along the

127

span of 3.5 billion years. Recently a list of 100,000 species of orchids has been reported. We are able to enjoy these creatures that are here with us, because they followed an evolutionary path slower than ours.

Which are the *controls* that determine the diversified manner in which the Creation evolves? A question never raised. To judge by the number of different evolutionary rates, the number of such controls should be incalculable and according to this theory equal to the number of *elemental particles and orders* ever evolved in the Creation.

Sociability and selectivity are essential requirements for the formation of any *order*. Because *order* reigns in the present Universe of systems *at all times,* it shall be accepted that *social drives* and *selectivity,* including that of *when* to associate, are essential to *all systems.* This power of *when* to associate is the only explanation of the unequal rate of evolution in the Universe that ultimately rests in the *freedom of decision* of all physical reality. The *unequal rate of evolution* definitively indicates that *association of systems* is *not deterministic* but freely exercised.

The argument can now be made, that the *essential* characters of reality are not embodied in the mere *process of association* when the associates have no input on it. Nor does this process justify the selective social drive of systems. Those characters shall be

embodied and **arise** from elemental matter and energy that are the agents and real components of the association. Thus *matter and energy in their most elemental state -unreachable to detection- shall be free, social and selective* as already argued in the previous Chapters II and III.

Every progressive level of evolution gives more complex systems and also more numerous ones, for complexity makes possible more arrangements. Protons, electrons and neutrons, three particles in total, yield 105 atoms. These atomic systems are more complex and more numerous than the previous three particles. The next level of evolution, the molecular world, counts with far more than one million compounds. More building blocks than the atoms have at their disposal allows the construction of millions of molecules from the simplest ones with two atoms to the very complicated ones with hundreds of them.

Between subsequent evolutionary strides the differences also widens, like *a system of umbrellas* where one shall cover the preceding one. Each umbrella ought to have a bigger radius and as a result the *increases* of their areas are greater and greater. With every evolutionary jump the creation busts its strength to surpass its previous jumps with increasing rates of improvements. A clear example is that of creatures' intelligences. Man is far more intelligent than the monkey. Down the evolutionary line the differences of intelligence are less and less noticeable. In sum, each successive evolutionary jump is more spectacular than the previous ones producing more spectacular systems and related functions. It is by reason and *by need* that the advancements should greatly supersede the previous accomplishments for functional faculties must control and therefore excel *all* previous ones. The reader may ask: If this is true, why don't we fly better and faster than birds? Or have better sensorial abilities than animals? My answer is that such abilities might be dormant, atrophied or under control of superior ones. In any case, I will not be surprised that one day some scientist will discover how to motorize properly a few atoms in our body to travel through air without the help of airplanes. There is plenty of energy available for this and more in the atomic world. Such energy had been tapped. The destructive capacity of the Hydrogen bomb is based on the release of a fraction of the nuclear bonds-energy of which we have trillions in our own cells.

THE ATOMIC WORLD.

The total mass gathered in a celestial body determines its class. By decreasing mass there are deemed to be stars, planets, satellites, meteorites, asteroids.., etc. Physical as well as chemical characters and the very life span of stars depend on the amount of mass. The reason is expressed by the Newton Formula

F= M x M'/k x d^2 where F is the gravitational force between M and M' masses, d is their distance and K is a constant depending on the media. All that is in the star is related to the internal energies created by gravitational forces and these in turn are related to its mass. Let's take an example, the Sun. It weighs almost one thousand times the weight of its nine planets. For this reason it is a star. Its composition is a mixture of H (Hydrogen) and He (Helium) nuclei because forces that correspond to its mass are able to trigger the nuclear reactions required to produce He nuclei from H nuclei but are not strong enough to produce more complex nuclei. The Sun's typical luminosity is due to the energy released in the H and He nuclei reactions and the gravitational waves. Every other character of the Sun: gravity at the surface, local densities, temperatures, pressures.., etc, are consequences of the same, its mass, its network of gravitational attractions and energies thereof derived.

Temperatures and pressures needed to produce other nuclei are found in the Supernovae, stars equivalent to 10^6 to 10^8 Suns. Explosions of these Superstars liberate the nuclei of most atoms. It is believed that our planetary system was formed out of the cosmic dust and debris ejected by the explosion of a Supernova -Sun

B- much greater than the Sun. Gradually such blasted materials concentrated by gravitational attraction and consolidated into planetary formations. Sun B proved to have done a thorough atomic production of atomic nuclei for, if not on other planets, on Earth we at least got the entire atomic world.

Places and processes of fabrication of atomic nuclei did not change with time. All nuclei were and still *are* created in the stellar kingdom, more complex ones in heavier and more energetic stars. The stars with their fierce temperatures and formidable pressures are the proper environments to generate the nuclei of the Periodic Table out of elemental matter. *Atomic nuclei,* then and now, become *atoms* if conditions drastically temper, and this occurs after stellar explosions when nuclei are released to unpressed spaces at freezing temperatures. There matter proceeds to form molecular structures. The evolutionary step of atoms to molecules in the microworld corresponds to another cosmic stride in the astroworld: the creation of non-ştellar formations, *the planets*, whose number and features are matter of speculation due to the lack of information we have concerning our planetary system.

To follow the evolution of systems we shall abandon the stars whose evolutionary levels are about the lowest in the Creation. Here on Earth we have the greatest evolutionary display from the bottom of inorganic materials up to the apex of organization, man. There are no other alternatives. Aside from the stars radiations we know close to nothing of other celestial bodies as planets and satellites. They are less powerful emitters of radiation and thus their messages get lost on their way to Earth. Access if possible would be too costly.

Let's start the exploration.

First take notice. No atomic element can be identified as such in our planet. Except for a few, the Noble Elements, the rest are unrecognizable. They have been buried in molecular structures where their atomic properties are totally concealed and overcome by molecular ones. (A similar reason to why man does not fly as do some of his ancestors). It may strike you to know that the Periodic Table was not completed until 50 years ago and the very existence of the atom was in question at the beginning of the century. Earth is a *molecular world* and diving into the atomic depths was a daring contemporary adventure.

Second surprise. The atoms percentage in terrestrial materials radically differ from those in the entire cosmos. That is an extremely unpredictable finding when we think that the Earth originated and is immersed in the Universe. How could it be so different to its surroundings? Evidently our planet is very odd, extremely *selective* or very privileged...to say the least. And fortunately for us such rarity will allow to follow the complete path of evolution.

Now, thanks to these recent discoveries I will be able to sketch for you the atomic edifices and to give a succinct idea of how atoms were uplifted to molecular components.

Protons and *neutrons* under the compression forces of the Supernova shortened their distances to a rage below 10^{-23} cm. where the *strong forces* erupted and welded themselves permanently into nuclei. Extraordinary amounts of energy were released in the bonding. Strong forces among two protons are 10^{39} times their gravitational pulling. No energy in the cosmos interfere with nuclear bonds for in order to break them it would be necessary to restore the amount of energy released when bonding, an impossible deed under earthly standards. After atomic nuclei are expelled in the Supernova explosion, nuclear particles do not separate again. Conversely these compact positive charged nuclei were able to fish *electrons* in number equal to their protons. Thus, electrical charges were neutralized and the *atomic structures* were completed not randomly but restricted to exquisite electronic designs. These are the blocks of which molecules are made of and the units that undergo transposition and combination in the course of chemical reactions. Each of the 105 elements or atoms is a distinct system with strict social order. Besides spatial organization no two electrons in a single atomic edifice are in the same energetic state.

The electronic organization in the atom has been precisely mapped and it appears to be specifically regulated. Electrons occupy energetic levels named orbital K, L, M, N, O, P, and Q, with capacities for 2, 8, 16, 32.., etc, electrons respectively.

Hydrogen, symbol H, the first element of the Periodic Table accommodates its *one* electron in orbital K. Helium, He, the second also fills the orbital K with its *two* electrons. Lithium, Li, the third has *three* electrons, two go to the level K and the third to level L. The seven following elements Beryllium, Boron, Carbon, Nitrogen, Oxygen, Fluorine and Neon (symbols Be, B, C, N, O, F, Ne) have two electrons in orbital K and the rest on orbital L. After level N is completed by the Ne's electrons, Sodium, Na, with *eleven* electrons fills K with two, L with eight and the remaining one settle on M orbital. And so on.

The electronic capacity of the orbital can be expressed by

$C = 2 \times N^2$, N being the number of the orbital. Thus:

K= 2 x 1^2 =2

L= 2 x 2^2 =8

M= 2 x 3^2 =18

N= 2 x 4^2 =32

O=...

P=...

Observe that as the capacities increase from 2, to 8, to 16, to 32, the increments 6, 8, 16 are greater and greater responding to the *umbrella effect* described previously.

Whereas nuclear configurations were set forever, the electronic atomic edifices were not. They had been affixed under weaker conditions and less energy was released in their bonding. To liberate them would not require a great effort. Electrons circulate around the nucleus at considerable distances solely held by electrostatic forces. These forces are weaker and when the distances of electrons to the nucleus increase they encourage socialization with other atoms' electrons. In fact, such is the unavoidable tendency of those electrons located in the outer orbitals. Social drives and new bondages of these outer electrons, the valences, overcome the ostracism of the previous atomic set up giving place to the next evolutionary level, *the molecular world.*

CHEMICAL INTERRELATIONS : THE VALENCES.

Electronic orbits enjoy stability when completed to full capacity. When they are not, the electron resort to *association* as the tool for a more stable situation. And another *innovation* springs up: the valence, the bond of molecular structures and voilá, Chemistry is born!

These new social links, valences, are the transfer or sharing of electrons between two atoms with the finality, it is said, to improve orbital stability. Don't miss here that *a purpose* is sought! This goal is achieved in several ways. Let's start with the case of Na (Sodium) and Cl (Chlorine). Their external orbitals present disparate configurations. Na has a single electron. Cl has seven. The orbital of Cl has capacity for 8. By transferring the Na's electron to the Cl's orbital, Na remains with a complete outer shell, the underlying one is electronically satiated with two electrons and not inclined to any social exchanges. Cl fills its outer orbital with the added electron. By this mechanism both atoms acquire the sought after orbital stability. But because the electron carries one negative charge the Cl become negatively charged while the Na is left positively charged by the loss of its electron. Now there is an electrical attraction that unites Na and Cl into a molecule NaCl, common salt. The chemical marriage had been accomplished entirely by the electrons' social activity.

This type of association is typical of inorganic compounds. Atoms of organic products associate through a different electronic interplay: the co-valence. C (Carbon) and H (Hydrogen) are the fundamental elements of organic products. CH_4 is the simplest organic construction. How is CH_4 bound?

C has four electrons in the outer orbital whose capacity is of eight. H has only one electron in an orbital capable of two. The covalent bondage can be visualized as two electrons, one from H and the other from C, being *shared* by both atoms. The H orbital has improved its stability by having *two shared* electrons, which also are enjoyed by C. As C has made the same type of connections with three other atoms of H its orbital has improved its energetic status with the *eight shared* electrons. At the close-to-light speed that electrons travel many amazing things happen that are unfamiliar to us, perhaps one of these is the happiness to share *permanently*. The positions of the electrons are not easily discernible and it may well be that the sharing or change in route of the electron does not have the significance that we are used to give to those events. Instead energy should be the prominent factor to deal with in the microworld. This theory sees the bond as a quantitative and qualitative *increase of energy* over that of the elements bonded and maybe the atoms see it as a benefit. Neighbors may see a benefit in sharing gardening tools. Is the increase of energy efficiency the reason of evolution?

There are other types of chemical valences that we will not go into, which further illustrate that molecular links are responsible for this evolutionary progress from the atomic to the molecular organization. What shall be emphasized is that contrary to expectations, the craving for association did not stop by satiating atomic orbitals with the bond of valences and formation of initial molecules. Once the orbits of all atoms were fulfilled the reason for atomic unrest had ended. In fact, at the solidification of the Earth's crust almost all matter was molecular, orbitals were stabilized. Nevertheless, the final resting equilibrium was not reached. Nothing could end the social thirst of matter, neither the aggressiveness nor inventiveness of evolution. Striking as it looks, socialization was more powerful than ever before and renewing itself at an accelerated pace. (The umbrella effect is in action where increments are greater and greater at each step up). Simple small molecules grew in complexity and size. Atomic elements were able to breed thousands of compounds in a staggering competition of adventurous associations witnessing the appearance of new properties and functions that culminated in the miracle of *life*.

This was not the end. Not at all, but rather the start of a brilliant evolutionary course towards the creation of man. *There is no end to creation*. This thesis tries to elucidate this fact.

NEW ORDERS. NEW CREATURES.

When matter or physical realities *spontaneously* associate they do it in an orderly fashion and the creation of a new order originates a new *identity*, a genuine creation, a new being without associates losing their *individualities*.

Two examples, crystallization and insects' societies will illustrate the point. These two examples have been chosen because the *individual* components remain unchanged within the association thus offering dramatic evidence that the novel properties evolved. Hence, the new emerging *identity*, relate directly to the association. In essence, *identity* arises from the whole structure of interrelations. From it derives its powers that are superior to those of any of the associated members or the accumulation of them when not properly interrelated. (The new identity carries the *evolved essences* of the elemental components: freedom of decision and capability to make meaning out of information.)

CRYSTALS.

When crystals are well developed they are striking visions of solid order, luminously enhanced by dazzling transparencies. Although their atoms are in continuous vibration, the crystal appears to the naked eye as a hard geometrical figure spatially symmetrical. The perfect picture of ordered association. It is not often that we come across well formed crystals, although *all solids have crystalline organization,* the atoms and molecules arranged along privileged directions.

Glass, despite its apparent solidity, is not considered a solid because its molecules are not placed in an orderly manner. They are too bulky, too irregular and move with difficulty in the molten state. When liquefied glass solidifies by cooling, its molecules get trapped in disorderly positions without time to form crystalline structures. And so glass is regarded as a *rigid liquid* rather than a solid. However, the capability of crystallization is there for crystals of glass have been obtained throughout laborious cycling of melting and cooling. One proof that to produce order is a capability of matter and an exigency of natural *spontaneous* association. Such *spontaneity* has been denied to glass. Order is the general status of physical reality.

Crystals are obtained by cooling molten materials as metals or by growing them from the concentrated solutions of their chemicals. In either method the free ions from atoms or molecules shall consecutively -so to speak- guess, search, travel, circumvent obstacles and find a final *resting* place (*dwelling* is a better word for they never rest) in the crystal formation. Like well trained soldiers! It is the materialization of crystalline *order* that ultimately earns the title of *solid state*. The strong agitation of atoms and molecules in the liquid state shall subside to a more subtle vibratory mood they enjoyed when encased in the crystal lattices. But before that happens, they diligently tuned into the direction that will bring them to their organized dwelling. The faces of the crystal usually grow steadily flat, sometimes when bathed by unequal concentration of material in different sections. Evidently the sections favored with greater density of materials shall exert less pulling over the materials than the other ones. How do they determine such forces? The mutual pulling forces among crystal and particles in the solution are *not gravitational forces* therefore not determined by their masses.

At what point such specific *crystalline drives* awake in those ionic swimmers? What forces *conceived* the *order* of the solid? How can the differences of these forces be explained? There are no answers to these questions and yet the entire surface of the Earth is crystalline matter. Invisible bits of pulverized materials made-up of hundreds of layers of tiny atoms (diameters of atoms are approx. 2 to 5 Angstroms) compactly deposited side by side. A crystal as small as 1cc. contains 2.5×10^{22} to 10×10^{22} atoms depending on its composition.

Several crystallographers of the last century independently systematized all crystal forms into 32 symmetry groups, which embrace the 230 types of possible crystals.

Again in crystals we face the *selectivity of form* that are reduced to a discrete number of crystal shapes 230, which become further reduced at the level of crystallographic *units* *to* 6.

Just as bricks build an edifice, the crystal grows by repetition of a *unit cell,* the building block that represents the unit pattern of the crystal. There are only six different building blocks, with them all crystals are made up, each growing up in one single type of block. (The umbrella effect in action. The increment from 1 molecule to 6 unit cells is 5. Those 6 unit cells are able to produce 230 different crystals. The increment 224 is much bigger than 5). The *unit cell* is an imaginary construction delineating the smallest arrangement of atoms that repeats itself along the various directions of the crystal. Frequently it encloses the atoms of the chemical formula. The building blocks shall fit together perfectly, and lined-up by tight juxtaposition they form the whole crystal. The flatness of the faces, the sharpness of angles, the total geometrical shapes are but a reflection of the internal *order* of the blocks.

In view of the architectonic blocks, the crystals are grouped into six systems: *Cubic, Tetragonal, Orthorhombic,*

143

Monoclinic, Triclinic and Hexagonal corresponding to the style of block used in the crystalline edifice.

We will not go into the detailed description of this glaring world of crystals except to point out the emergence of the *identity crystal,* an evolutionary innovation with new qualities and powers not contained in the atoms or in the unit cells. And to indicate the role that such *identity* plays in the genesis of crystalline organization.

CRYSTAL'S PROPERTIES AND CONTROL.

Organized matter has properties unseen in unorganized matter. The uplifting from amorphous form to crystal, as from sound to symphony, is the success of organization.

In the making of a crystal the forces that tie together the atoms are weaker than the chemical bonds, the valences, holding atoms into molecules. A simple percussion that breaks the crystal has no effect whatsoever on the molecular bonds. Consequently the crystalline organization, by not interfering with chemical relations, do not alter properties related to chemical composition while adding new ones due to the atoms' distribution in the crystal and crystallographic links.

That some of the properties such as elasticity depend on the distribution is evident because identical values of these properties are repeated along parallel arrays whereas such values change in other directions. Similarly mechanical, thermal, electrical, magnetic and optic properties are conditioned to the internal order. For instance, a typical behavior of crystals is *cleavage*. A crystal cleaves uncovering perfect flat faces along those planes where crystallographic bondages are the weakest. Some crystals have several *planes of cleavage*.

It is to the *crystal* that such properties are attached, not to the components either singled or disorderly amassed.

The *crystal* controls its growth, the cooperation of the whole structure, the total coordination of functions that is patent in the right positioning of atoms. When corners and edges grow disproportionately faster than planes developing rare shapes, the exact equal shapes develop in all symmetrical regions. Snow flakes exemplify such ostentatious growths, all identical in *six directions.* How do atoms in one corner know and copy *simultaneously* the arrangements of the other five? Or vice versa? Simply, *they don't*, because no atom or corner has the proper information to do it, unless they are under *control* of the *new identity*: the crystal. The crystal is in command with the power to process the information of the whole system.

Instant spontaneous change of structure is another marvel of coordinated action. There are compounds that may adopt several crystallographic forms, some more stable than others at certain temperature. Silicon dioxide is one of them. Changing the temperature we may witness a sudden metamorphosis of the crystal from one crystallographic form to another one. What accounts for the *unanimous* moving of atoms to a new *unrehearsed* order? It is obvious that a single atom is comfortable in its position at both ranges of temperatures and not aware of either formation. It is the crystal edifice that is *not*, and so it controls and changes the positions of its atoms.

One last experiment to endorse this view. Sodium chlorate crystallizes in two forms: dextrogiro and levogiro. The first deviates the polarized light towards the right, the second towards the left. The solution of sodium chlorate has no effect in polarized light . Either form can be obtained by placing in the solution a *seed* crystal of sodium chlorate, if this is dextrogiro so it will be the resulting crystal and viceversa. The chlorate and sodium ions populating the solution are indifferent to either structure. That seed, dextrogiro or levogiro, will determine what form to grow. It imposes its control *on the process to associate* to satiate its energetic needs, and on the crystal's growth to secure its stability.

In short. The crystal is a new *identity* with new characters that none of its components had.

SOCIAL SYSTEMS.

Identities are the controllers of their established orders and although they are not sensorially perceived their physical effects are plainly detectable even in associations of clearly separate individuals.

Organization does not come to a halt at reaching our familiar dimensions of living creatures. Indeed the sociability of creatures, if synchronized into a *unified order*, such *construction* can be classed as an *identity*.

Inferior creatures in their associations closely resemble the atoms in a crystal. Atoms are incapable of appreciating the beauty of the clear castle they made. Likewise insects are bound to and unaware of the wisdom of their colony, whose character and functions transcend those of the individual insect.

Let's turn our attention to the fascinating happenings going on within one of these social groups: the beehive.

The hive is a pool of activity, an ancestral organism that through the ages has adapted the very morphology of the bees to the effectiveness of their labors, as cells in living creatures do differentiate according to bodily functions. There are generally three types of bees: the queen, one for each hive, several thousands workers occasionally reaching up to 30,000, and a few drones. The hive consists of wax curtains with hundreds of fluted rooms to host eggs or honey. Compressed by their own weight, the rooms become hexagonal shaped.

The queen deposits one egg on each of these hexagonal cells while she is fed and licked constantly by the workers. She is practically an egg-machine pouring 4 to 5 thousand eggs a day, during 4 or 5 years. By contrast the life of the drones is very short. They fly with the queen in her first and only flight. One of them fertilizes her and at her return to the hive she sheds off her wings and devotes herself to incessant procreation. Drones are eliminated when food is scarce for their job is finished.

Workers take over the rest of the tasks, which are prolific and sophisticated. For one: the manufacturing of honey. Bees have the exclusive secret of the whole process. There is no artificial, no man-made honey. From the taking of pollen, the concentration of it that they do by *ventilation* beating their wings, to the end product, every detail is scrupulously carried out by the workers. To produce one pound of honey bees made 36,000 trips to gather pollen and the factory is kept continuously clean, for the slightest odor will spoil the honey. The bee flies beating its wings 200 times for second. This requires energy, more so with the burden of carrying pollen back home. It is not surprising that in one month the bee, too exhausted to reach home will fall to the ground and die.

The feeding and caring of larvae is another demanding job. Each egg hatches in three days and from then on the larvae should be fed and cleaned once *every minute*. Their diet is rigorously strict: two days of royal jelly and the next four pollen mix with honey. If it is a queen larvae, she is served another diet heavier in royal jelly. On the seventh day they start threading silky cocoons and the workers build a wax door closing the cell that will be opened by the new bee in 12 days. Later comes the instructing of the infant bees.

In between these tasks, there is the continuous transmission of information through the typical dances indicating the location of food, the constant licking of exuded chemicals peculiar to each beehive, the distribution of food to colony guests from whom bees derive some benefit, and the defense of the hive.

A bee isolated from the beehive has no chance of survival. In it the bee operates, lives and dies subordinating its own individuality to the reasons and life of the beehive. When bees attack enemies of the colony, they must know that once the sting is in, they will not be able to pull it without being torn apart and die. But they do not hesitate and do not lack courage in the charge. Is this a voluntary act or are they controlled by the hive? If so under what conditions do these controls work? Answers to these questions may open a door to brilliant discoveries in three human transcendental fields: genetic medicine, rehabilitation programs and social reforms, as we will explore at the end of this thesis.

The hive activities are not incompetent, superfluous or accidental. They are perfectly coordinated, meaningful and accurately executed from the familiar routines to the complicated and peaceful splitting of the hive in two kingdoms when a new queen is born. The uniqueness of the event makes no difference. No confusion, no quarrels, no war. A clever social program!

Wasps, ants, termites live harmonically in similar societies. The collective behavioral resources are numberless, perfectly orchestrated, a truly *spontaneous* government including curious expressions of slavery-practices, heroic deeds, organization of labor, war strategies, storage and preservation of food.

The colony is a higher structural order above that of the members, where all proceed in *unison*, freely done, even when self denial is required. The informational load is *endowed* to the *identity of the system* in its natural assemblage of vitalistic relations.

Insect mechanisms have been described, energy consumed in the processes have been estimated, codes

150

of communication translated, morphological diversities reconciled with functional specialties, *but* the *source of the program* that precisely and tenaciously governs the colonies is inaccessible to present scientific comprehension. It belongs to the realm of the unknowable, the realm of the *new identity*, the new creature: *the colony*.

No man-made honey! It is the secret of the *hive*.

CHAPTER VII. - EARTH

Earth emerges as a packed cosmic cloud of material fairly distinct and isolated from its surroundings about 7 billion years ago. After the accretion of the masses the development during the next 3 billion years is quite obscure. There is no contributing data that can tell the story of the organization and structuration of our planet. Rocks keep records of these early events, and no rocks have been found beyond 3.5 billion years back. Information from meteorites, whose origin is supposed to be terrestrial or those coming from the moon, covers the same period of time.

The Earth's core according to contemporary studies does not differ greatly from its earlier state. Presently, it is still liquid, and temperatures rising towards its inner center may well reach 4,000° K. These harsh conditions and the untaming energies to be endured prevent the evolvement of systems that otherwise richly flourish on the surface. Thus, keeping on the trail of the evolvement of systems we must turn our attention towards the solid crust and the atmosphere, which are the elements that foster, quicken and participate in the workings of evolution.

The date of the crust's solidification has been debated from many points of view from consideration of the content of salt in the oceans to analysis of geological and anthropological findings and reasoning on the principle of energy conservation. The estimates given, that started a few thousand years ago, were inadequate. Short a few hundred million years. Although successively these figures had been enlarged, not until the discovery of radioactivity in 1895, had the issue been settled. Under this new light previous studies have been reviewed. With the help of radioactive materials, whose reliability in terms of time clock is conclusively proven, the solidification of the crust has been placed at about 4.5 billion years ago. The official birth of the planet is definitively set at that time.

ATMOSPHERE AND SURFACE OF THE EARTH.

Earth is gifted with an atmosphere. It is not the general case. Some planets have atmospheres and others do not, a fact that is related to the planet's mass for atmosphere exists where gravitational forces are able to retain one. This is the sole reason why the Earth, with gravity six times stronger than the moon, still has one, while the latter, a smaller formation, has been depleted of what could have been, if ever it had, its original atmosphere.

Gravitational forces also affect the composition of the atmospheres. By inertia the components of any gaseous mixture move at different speeds. The lightest ones are faster runners. In the particular case of atmospheres, massive gases are more firmly held by gravity than those with lighter mass, and when molecules reach the velocity of escape, which for Earth is 7.1 miles/sec., they may engage in space traveling without serious opposition. Throughout this process the total composition gradually alters and it could radically change along a wide span of time.

In comparison the crust, because it is solid, has a relative permanency despite the chemical influences of the atmosphere upon every substance it contacts. Reactions with CO_2 produce carbonates, Nitrogen develops nitrates and nitrogen compounds, and Oxygen and Hydrogen oxidizes and hydrates respectively a high percentage of terrestrial products.

The initial gaseous outer layer of the atmosphere was predominantly a mixture of H_2, NH_3, CH_4 and H_2O all immediate combinations of Hydrogen with other atoms and certainly the gases to be expected from a Universe made almost entirely of Hydrogen. The reader may remember that the sources of solids and complex atoms were the Supernovae, makers and containers of every nuclei of the Periodic Table. In their explosion nuclei were ejected and atoms and molecules were formed.

Hydrogen, being the lightest component of the atmosphere, it quickly went to the exosphere, the outermost layer of it. There H_2 was bombed by the UV radiation of the Sun and steadily energized to higher and higher speeds until the gravity was unable to retain it and inevitably sooner or later plunged into space. Heavier elements, in order to increase their speeds consume more energy and therefore are left behind.

As of today the largest planets: Uranus, Saturn, Neptune, and Jupiter have atmospheres of lighter gases than Earth including Hydrogen because they are giant planets and their gravity grasp is more powerful. Since their very beginnings they were able to control their *total* atmospheres preventing it from escaping.

Subtle halos circle the bigger planets while heavier mixtures of gases circle less massive ones if they have an atmosphere at all. The Universe is made out of contrasts!

It is very possible that our planet totally dissipated its *first atmosphere* when it was in the molten state, if such was once its state. Discordant opinions on the subject, however, agree on one fact: that the Earth was an *extremely hot* place at the time. It was radiating plenty of energy coming in from various sources. Radioactivity was 15 times greater than at present. In the process of growing, Earth was still incorporating solids to its total mass, being constantly struck by meteorites, rocks and other cosmic materials trapped in its gravitational field. It was actually roasting under an implacable Sun. The gaseous shell was not a protection against the scorching solar UV radiation, which is mitigated today by the ozone absorption taking place in the periphery. That primordial atmosphere was perfectly transparent to the full spectrum of solar radiation. Presently the surface temperature is below $100C^0$ bouncing in an interval of 100 degrees. The thermosphere from 80 to 480 kilometers above the Earth have a range of temperature increasing from about -90^0 C to about 1500^0 C. Initially, temperatures were of the order of 10^5 K degrees from top to bottom. That is unimaginable hot. (Kelvin degrees are equal to Centigrade plus 273 for 0^0 Kelvin is equal to 273^0 Centigrade. Thus, $100,000°$ K is practically $100,000°$ C).

It is believed that at a certain point in time, fantastic amounts of H and CO were ejected from internal layers as today still are by volcanoes, supplying the planet with a *new atmosphere*. Although calm was restored, temperatures continued to rise because CO_2 and O_2 mixed together bar the passage of infrared rays.

They actually acted as a natural greenhouse reflecting down the heat emitted by the crust, which turned into a burning plate. Waters in contact with it steamed furiously, forming clouds of such size and density that no light could penetrate them. Earth was in a permanent closed dark night.

Instead, the clouds were illuminated and *hit* by persistent solar radiation that split H_2O into H^+ and OH^-, and that then provoked the next dissociation of OH^- into more and very active $O^=$. This ion now displaced H from the CH_4 and NH_3 molecules. Simultaneously with the chemical reactions, the electricity carried by the ions was charging the clouds. When overcharged to explosive extremes, they bursted in monumental lightnings and torrential rains of incredible intensity and duration. That is how the oceans were formed. When oceans appeared, temperatures fell below the boiling point of water in most part of the planet. Hundred of years of rain mitigated land and skies. Water became the dominant element of the Earth.

After clouds had vanished, sunlight was permitted to illuminate the globe. A blue layer of ozone was being generated by the very active $O^=$ and it started to abate the rigors of the solar UV rays. Meanwhile Oxygen was entering the scene in small but consistent amounts. An *oxygenated atmosphere* was timidly breaking its path.

Earth had finally established a new phase of control. Violence had been tempered and molecular association made possible. Now that the process of organization was protected, the spring of life -*the new invention of evolution*- was, as always had previously been a *new social gathering of matter*. It bloomed at every opportunity for energy was there, tamed but inherent, as aggressive as ever but *channeled* to express its activity in new forms, new controls, new orders and new systems.

At this juncture the narrative is open to many questions to which there are no definitive answers. The length of the evolving eras cannot be ascertained with accuracy nor can the extend and exactness of the processes. One thing is sure that the first manifestations of life were necessarily *anaerobic* for no O_2 was available. Recent research has proven that high complex biosystems in the depth of oceans are supported by Sulfur derivatives without any help of O_2. Therefore, life might have appeared under different biomechanisms than the ones currently seen on Earth.

By space considerations most life should have been lodged in the oceans that cover more than 3/4 of the planet. In addition, the medium water itself offers a number of advantages, friction protection, free movement, heat shelter., etc.

It was not until 2 to 2.5 billion years ago that the Earth was endowed with an *oxidizing atmosphere*.

The transition from the first, a *reducing one*, to its full substitution was a painfully slow interchange of elements that perhaps never would have been completed without the advent of green plants which brought along *revolutionary innovations:* the creation of organic matter and the production of free Oxygen in overwhelming amounts...at the tiny cost of visible light. Plants changed the atmosphere and the face of the Earth.

The *oxidizing atmosphere* was a most *rare* gift. Rare, because the exclusivity of the phenomenon, and the donor, the green plants. Only the green ones extract from light the energy to split CO_2 in the most extraordinary atoms of evolution: Carbon, the center piece of life, and Oxygen, the supporter of it...at large. Rare, because an oxidizing atmosphere is a singular event in the known Universe. Rare, because its spectacular results. It accelerated evolution to its highest peaks in *no time* compared with the previous cosmic evolution of earthy inorganic materials.

LIFE.

Scarcely half a century ago Chemistry was divided in Inorganic and Organic. The first dedicated to products of the inanimate world, the second to those constituting living organisms which could not be synthesized for an essential ingredient was not available in the lab: *life.*

The separation wall proved to be built in sand. In 1928 an organic compound, *urea,* was obtained by the simplest of techniques, heating inorganic materials. During the following 75 years the number of synthetic organic products had surpassed by far the total number of chemicals produced by then since the beginning of the alchemy. *Organic Chemistry* became downgraded to the *Chemistry of Carbon* for Carbon was present in *all* organic molecules.

Still to this day complex living processes are being treated with reverence for *life* keeps its mysterious presence. It is implicitly accepted that living creatures have faculties whose province lay in the field of religion and emotions beyond the reach of scientific analysis. Those beliefs are retained because the reluctance of science to incorporate non-tangible realities as a proper matter of scientific studies, a self-inflicted wound in the inquiry of the nature of reality.

The differences between high organized living beings and inorganic matter are certainly striking. But on the line of less and less complex systems those differences become less and less conspicuous. The *umbrella effect* explains that the increment of these differences increases at every step up on the evolutionary ladder.

Therefore, it is not surprising that life in its higher manifestations appear to be a sudden miracle not grounded in the potential of elemental matter.

Life for highly organized systems entails living functions: capacity of reproducing their kind *spontaneously*, control over their surroundings and ability to compel permanent changes in structure, which are transmitted to the next generation. These familiar features in higher creatures are somehow fuzzy at the borders of the simplest forms of life. Viruses, for instance, *duplicate* themselves although with the help of cells that they must invade. And *replication* is the only exponent of life they have.

Perhaps what is needed is a more complete and appropriate definition of *life*. Nonetheless it is obvious that sometime in the development of our planet *life* must have had a beginning.

How do our chemists cross the bridge from molecular matter on primitive Earth to the springs of life? And, what *organic* compounds should be set aside as *non-living* matter in the up lifting evolvement of life?

To this effect a series of experiments have been conducted simulating the original conditions of the planet. Mixtures analogous to the first and second atmospheres have been subjected to the action of various physical agents: electrical sparks, heat up to 1,000C°, bright sun light, UV rays, ultrasonic vibrations, gamma rays.., etc. Scientists discovered that the mix of CH_4, NH_3, and H_2 representing the *first atmosphere* gives more varied and richer quantities of organic molecules than the second one. Several days of electrical sparks over the reducing mixtures resulted in a large and diversified deposit of organic compounds, some of them were the building blocks of the proteins that are essential to life.

Although recently beams of electrons activated by the cyclotron also compete for the successful results, it is still reasonable to conclude that the first atmosphere originated a great percentage of organic products. The boost to the second atmosphere was precisely given by the profusion of green plants that had been produced not only by organic materials but also *by huge amount of them.* Before vegetation spread, quantities of O_2 must have been very low and therefore a poor support of organic production. Our best bet relies on the first reducing atmosphere.

A step beyond had been attempted with experiments geared to reproduce the *spontaneous* formation of proteins. By heating a mixture of aminoacids it was expected that a permanent dehydratation would occur. A peptide is basically a chain of 20 to about 30 aminoacids. The experiment was effectively carried on and after cooling some peptides links had been formed. The loss of water among the molecules had caused the bondage. Proteins are not so far away for basically they are bigger molecules usually containing more than 50 aminoacids linked together.

These processes could be the ones that might have occurred during centuries of violent storms in the heavy atmosphere covering the whole planet. Aminoacids falling from the rain in the hot crust and there suffering dehydratation and linkage. Later these peptides might have been swept to the oceans by torrential waters where clement conditions were assured and hence the lasting of large molecules.

The role of proteins in the living world is very important and specific. There are actually *precise* messages determining biological activities. To explain the significance of these messages let's assign one symbol to each of the 24 exclusive aminoacids that regularly appear in the proteins of biosystems. Just as our alphabet has 26 letters. (Some proteins have thousands of these symbols). An average protein containing about 500 is an unmistakable *word* in the biological language. We don't have any word with 500 letters. Items as complex and numerous as persons could be identified around the world with shorter numbers of symbols in a passport and background records.

That proteins could have been originated by *chance* is hereafter flatly excluded. There is no possibility to construct *one protein* containing 500 aminoacids of a particular class and in a particular order...by lottery. The number of potential arrangements is a figure like 1 followed by one to a few hundred zeros according to the calculations of noted scientists. The calculus of probabilities in which these estimates are based applies to situations of perfect disorder. This first requirement is already missed in any natural situation for none is in homogeneous disorder. But let's dismiss such *detail*. Eddington estimated the total number of elemental particles of the Universe to be 1 followed by 27 zeros. The reader shall be reminded that one additional zero reflects 10 times this amount, two zeros 100 times this amount and so on. That means that nothing less then 1 followed by several hundred zeros Universes will be needed to provide material for the arrangements of 500 aminoacids of which only one will be *the protein* sought. Assuming the portent granted, the protein produced, what will a single protein do in solitude and inauspicious surroundings? The appearance of life cannot be rooted in *one single* and rare incidence. Where in the Universe are all the other proteins alike or not alike to this one needed by all living creatures? The improbable reaches the absurd. The human body has about 50,000 more complex proteins than the *one* considered.

To the genesis of *that* protein shall be added the factor of time attached to chemical processes. Aminoacids shall collide to join each other to hit the right target. The possible arrangements above numbered to yield one acceptable protein will consume an unimaginable magnitude of time, trillions upon trillions the life span of the Creation. There was not such *fortunate* protein furthermore entrusted with the creation of every living creature on Earth in the scarce last billion years. *We cannot accept such a portent.*

The high specificity of organic compounds definitively precludes *cause by chance* as a serious thought. There are more rational agents that orchestrated their making. Experiments and observation have proven that even *if* the laws of chance are forced by inducing disorder, the course of *spontaneous* synthesis is not random and arbitrary. Take the case of polypeptides' synthesis. When a sufficient variety of monoacids are stimulated to react randomly, surprisingly and repeatedly the resulting peptides are few, always the same with every test, while a great number of others equally possible do not appear at all. There is an intelligent process at work that chooses ones with preference to others. Similar findings are obtained with regard to structure. If structural coils of proteins are randomly dispersed, when the dispersion action ceases, the proteins *spontaneously* recover their normal shapes. Notwithstanding that to remain random could be much easier. Intelligent mechanisms and controls were there continuously operating their development.

In short, there is no *chance* in the protein origin and production.

One sentence summarizes the importance of the proteins: life cannot exist without proteins. Proteins are recognized in the biological world for the type and number of atoms, the order of the aminoacids and their molecular structures. Even proteins identically equal but one having the atoms disposed as mirror-image to the other are discriminated by living organisms. All life is built on proteins L (levogiro), which are those that bend the plane of polarized light towards the left. The exact protein D (dextrogiro) that bends the polarized light to the right is systematically absent in living creatures except for extremely unusual occurrences. There is always room for the exception in a free universe as this thesis postulates. The Theory of Systems interprets our Universe as fundamentally free.

NUCLEI ACIDS AND LIFE.

Despite the extraordinary contributions to the phenomena of life, proteins are not yet the chemical answer to life for they do not have the ability to replicate. The answer is embodied in the nucleic acids known as DNA and RNA, which are molecules capable of self-replication and undergo changes (mutations) transmittable to their molecular replicas. These are the classic characters of life. Nucleic acids are the simplest living systems.

Nucleic acids are more complex and have molecular weights superior to that of proteins, on the average of 6,000,000 units. (The molecular weight unit is the weight of the Hydrogen atom). As proteins are chains of aminoacids, nucleic acids are chains of nucleotides. Each nucleotide contains three chemical groups: one phosphate, one sugar and a nitrogen compound (nitrogen base) that is laterally attached to the sugar. The chain backbone is made up of the phosphates and sugars while the nitrogen compounds hang along like side appendices. They are only four: adenine, thymine, guanine and cytosine, in DNA; and uracyl, guanine, adenine and cytosine in RNA.

The nucleic acids are named after their sugar that is Ribose in RNA (Abb. for Ribonucleic acid) and Deoxy Ribose in DNA (Abb. for Deoxy Ribo-nucleic acid.)

When describing the structures of the nucleic acids I will refer to DNA structure in preference to RNA because there is less information about the latter and, for another more important reason, DNA occupies a higher functional rank than RNA in cellular functioning. It presides over the synthesis of RNA and proteins, and carries the hereditary material of the species. While the RNA family (there are at least three structural different RNAs in each cell of highly organized creatures)

167

mainly synthesizes proteins following instructions of the DNA.

The great majority of the DNA molecules consists of two chains of nucleotides entwined around each other like a spiral staircase. The appendiced nitrogen bases fall inside and they attach among themselves by weak hydrogen bonds forming what could be visualized as the steps of the staircase.

The sugar-phosphate backbones, the two banisters of the stair, are exactly the same in all DNAs. Hence they do not carry any special information for any DNA. Instead the combinations of the four nitrogen bases differ from the DNAs of one specie to the DNAs of others, and they encode the instructions for the synthesis of products and cellular activity of a particular biosystem. The nitrogen bases are the carriers of information in the biological world.

The replication process of nucleic acids is simple, clean, efficient and it is accomplished in minutes. A virus can make several hundred replications in 20 minutes. The double helix separates both chains and each chain acts as a mold (template) attracting from the medium the molecules that are the same as the complement missed in the separation. It is obvious that the medium shall contain such molecules otherwise the replication fails for lack of supporting surroundings. Replication is done within living systems but can be done outside of them also in non-living systems (named free-cell cultures) when they are provided with: a) the nucleic acid to serve as template, b) adequate enzyme (protein that initiates or accelerates the reaction), and c) products needed in the construction of the chain.

The result of replication is the formation of two identical DNAs, which encompass the precise copy of atoms, order, distances, bonds, energies.., etc. If we name the chains A and B, chain-A will be complemented with a new chain-B. And chain-B will get the new complement chain-A. Thus, the two equal stairs are built.

Self-replication has some analogies with the mechanisms of the crystal growth in that the seed crystal extracts from the proper environment atoms and molecules *of its own kind* and organizes them into *its own structure.* Selective attraction, external control and organizational power are manifested in both processes, crystallization and self-replication. But sharp qualitative differences between the two processes are plain. Selectivity, control and organization reach a much higher level of sophistication when DNA is in charge. DNA alone, one single molecule (the seed of the crystal is a group of molecules) selects and controls very specific and complex molecules (those of the crystal are very simple ones) and creates the exact replica of self by chemical reactions (not by merely juxtaposition of particles in the lattices of the crystal as the seed crystal does).

The two DNAs, after replication, are totally independent and endowed with the same regulatory powers of the initial DNA, which comprehends: synthesis of a great variety and number of compounds, and triggering a sequence of cellular activities whose updated list is quite long and extraordinarily impressive, yet incomplete still in course of research. And those tasks are completed in a very short time, like every living action. In one word: DNA is alive. In comparison, the crystal merely provides *traffic control* and accommodation of atoms in the crystal by a painfully slow process. However it shall be accepted that crystallization is an incipient attempt of matter in the same direction of self-replication and it is an actual self-organization and neat exhibition of external control.

Returning to the subject of the origin of life. The high levels of exclusivity of nucleic acids' structures and functions further weaken the science position to attribute the origin of life to *chance*. The mechanisms of evolution ought to be universal and consistent because life is evolving along the same patterns every place at all times. Evolution does not rest in fortuitous, unrepeatable events are every evolutionary step in the micro and macro-world. At arriving at the stage of life, the staggering number of intelligent processes urgently demands the revision of the *essential* regulations of evolution.

How and where were nucleic acids invented? How did the supporting environment of life evolve? Biologists and chemists have joined efforts on these matters, the ones trying to adjudicate the evolving functions of life to the cellular system; the others restraining themselves to the evolvement of molecules up to the nucleic acids. The problem of life has finally obliged the blend of fields in the common ground of Biochemistry, a soundly justified discipline.

MEMBRANES AND NUCLEIC ACIDS.

As already mentioned, it is accepted that a great many organic compounds were synthesized on the terrestrial crust some 4 billion years ago and later washed into the oceans. Problems arise when it is questioned : How could these tiny molecules, invisible to the eye, maneuver their way from peptides to proteins? And more intricate yet: How has the assemblage of nuclei acids been accomplished?

Nucleic acids could not possibly evolve in the oceanic medium from incipient organic molecules without help. Organic products reaching the seas proceed from narrow bands of continental edges and they ought to have been in very small amounts. Dropped on immense and relentless waters, isolation was their sure fate. With absolute certainty it can be stated that *social forces* of such particles were ineffective in those large distances and against the strength of overwhelming currents. They could not associate and without association no evolution could ever come out.

Fortunately, water proved to be an ally of evolution. (This fact cannot surprise us because the whole Earth promotes evolution and water is 3/4 part of it). Water splits molecules into atoms or groups of atoms electrically charged: the ions. For instance, NaCl splits into Na^+ and Cl^-. Ions appeal to water that is electrically *asymmetric* (a dipole). Thus, a layer of concentrated water around organic matter could have sheltered clusters of them and the products enclosed within this shelter were prevented from wandering around. Social relations among the trapped molecules were now feasible because their distances have been reduced to a limited size and they stayed constantly within each others' reach. Frontiers established by such walls of water shelled the system and that made possible and protect its self-organization. With this, evolution had launched *another invention*: the membrane. This one, by defining a territory, paved the road for the evolvement of the cell viewed by biologists as the unit of life.

THE CELL.

The potential of organic matter to *spontaneously* segregate and to initiate membranic enclosures has already been triggered in the lab. Moreover, to induce such formations has been proven to be amazingly easy. Many different products under diverse circumstances render them. From solutions of large organic molecules have been observed the growing of conglomerates of matter that resemble a sort of pre-biological *enclosed* orders. These systems control to a certain extent the external surroundings from which they selectively extract molecules raising their inside concentration on occasions to thirty times that of the outside solution. Chemical reactions also proceed at a faster rate within themselves than the same reactions outside, apparently due to a peculiar control. These formations have been named *coacervates*.

More evolved yet are the *microspheres* that separate when hot solutions of peptides are cooled. Immediately the spherules display a distinct membrane and, in time, an internal granular organization. Some microspheres all of a sudden divide in two, as cells (amebae) do, without stimuli to account for; another *spontaneous* free decision. Others have been observed to swim in a non-random fashion contrary to scientific rules. There are functions going in those small systems that the medium does not have, and that can be aptly described as resulting from an organization, an intelligent one, a new *identity*.

Back to our topic. In the earlier times of our planet it seems improbable if not impossible that molecules without a supporting environment could have evolved life. Organic matter on the ardent surface of the Earth would have been burned in no time. On the seas, molecules, no matter how spherical and compact their structures would have been, were still too vulnerable when left alone in a ocean full of vigor and lack of understanding for organic needs. They probably would have been quickly destroyed or dispersed. Not so when protected by an envelope of *concentrated water*, in the case when a water molecule of the outer layer is dislocated, another from the surroundings will replace it without disturbing the internal components. Or, in the alternative, by buying time the whole spherule could escape, as spherules do, to peaceful locations where self-organization could germinate. Organic materials, thus, might have avoided the menace posed by giant elements using as a defense their very own tool: water. (It pays to be as wise as Nature is).

Now it is time for the hen-egg question: Which comes first, the nucleic acid or the membrane? Disregard how rudimentary any of them might have been at their origins. Need is the mother of invention. Let me say that no evolutionary invention sits idle waiting for another invention to appear and solve its problems. This Universe is not a lazy or obtuse one.

Regular membranes are formed in the lab at the peptide level but the water dipoles do not need such kind of sophistication to act and *water membranes* may have been formed at the *very first chemical opportunity*. More so the need for membranes to be a shelter in the seas than in the undisturbed lab cultures. All the more because the low cost and availability of water. Thus, it is my opinion that once peptides appear, and obviously before that, surely they were protected by a membrane that facilitated the subsequent evolvement of nucleic acids. Like everything else the membrane must have been perfected with time. Thus, membranes having appeared for simple organic matter, were in place, although subject to evolvement, at the advent of the highly sophisticated nuclei acids.

Let's reflect on the opposite. How did simple organic matter fight the impossible maritime battle to become high rank, complex and large nucleic acids without the help of membranes? And if successful, how do you convince this author that nucleic acids *decided* to fortify their organic dwellings with a membrane that had been available to peptides and other molecules long ago? Both propositions are unacceptable: to retain that nucleic acids *evolved* without help, and to ascribe them the task of creating the entire biosystem membrane included. In my opinion the evolvement of the nest, the envelope, the membrane, ought to have been a step ahead, in preparation for, and to facilitate the evolvement of the nucleic acids. We have seen these *anticipatory* insights to be a universal gift of Nature.

Nature does not work by inventing the *difficult* before the *easy*, and creating the *complex* to solve the *simple*. It works in comparable levels of order and organization. In short, the collective collaboration of Nature precludes a *chemical evolution* of life isolated from the *biological evolution* of it. That is, the creation of a *magic molecule* out of the evolutive context of the morphology and physiology of systems.

Probably next to the membrane a selective flux of materials in and out of the system might have developed corresponding to various chemical chain reactions not possible to coordinate in the open. Similar mechanisms also appear *spontaneously* in experimental formations. In any event, the novelty of the organic grouping under protective boundaries qualify as an *evolutionary design* in its way of becoming a cell. From now the membrane and the enclosed products would evolve as a system. Even today's DNAs, simplest as those of virus or highly complex, cannot function without support. Instead the opposite has been reported: that the removal of DNA from a cell does not bring immediate cellular death. Unicellular organisms may survive weeks without nucleus, where most of the DNAs reside, and cells of higher organisms last several months with appreciable regenerative powers, growth differentiation and production of proteins and enzymes. If nothing else, these are indications that life is not a linear process strictly chemical, but a system operation. The resilience of the membrane and other key elements are characteristic features that we identify with life. Thus, life is not the exclusive domain of the nuclei acids.

If DNA is alive because it can produce another DNA, so too are alive the primitive nucleotides or organic matter that eventually originated the DNA. All are expressions of an unfolding universal life: the life of systems.

COMMON ORIGEN OF LIFE REVISED.

The amount of DNA is constant in the cells of every creature and soon DNA was equated with the hereditary material of the species. Just as musical tapes convey precise notes of symphonies, likewise the DNA conveys the instructions for the living activities of the cell. In its structure is encoded the information required in the development of the whole creature. That is achieved by replications of DNA, cellular division, differentiation of tissues, formation of organs..

etc.., The extraordinary cellular diversification operated in the maturation of high organisms does not modify the structure of the DNAs. All DNAs contain the same information for it has been exactly transferred in the replication of DNA. It is proven by the fact that when a cell from a tissue is transplanted to another one it adapts to the new situation in shape and function becoming indistinguishable among its neighbors.

A gene is the region of DNA that instruct the synthesis of one protein.

DNA is a number of juxtaposed genes with a few nucleotides marking the end of a gene and the beginning of the next. Man has about one million proteins, hence about one million genes in the DNA. A virus may have from a few to several hundreds. Bacteria one thousand to several thousand.

Three nucleic pairs (three steps in the staircase of DNA) guide the formation of one aminoacid. To build a protein of 200 aminoacids, 600 nucleotide-pairs are needed.

The number of DNAs in each human cell is not known. Almost the totality of the DNA material is in the nucleus of the cell and when the cell divides it separates into formations called chromosomes. At least each one contains one DNA, for DNA does not break in the process. Then the minimum number of DNA molecules in man is 46.

The control of the DNA organization, even at high levels of complexity, is quite efficient and complete. As said above, DNA never falls apart spontaneously. Conversely, it forms spontaneously when the correct ingredients are present: the DNA-seed to guide the constructions of the replica and the medium with the proper material for it. This entails the opening of the double helix spontaneously, an actual breaking apart that does not occur except when anticipating replication.

Although each species has a particular sequence of nitrogen bases, the code is universal (allowing for exceptions) for all living creatures. That is, the language of the nitrogen bases is the same in all of them. On this basis it has been concluded that *all creatures have a common origin.* I agree with this conclusion although not in the argument, in the face of the specificity of the universe at the quanta level, and the specificity of the evolutive process. Neither offers but one alternative. Nature does not have two solutions for one problem. The code is one because it is the *only possibility* for evolution.

There are 105 atoms, no more, from here to the end of the Creation, because physical reality has no other atomic solutions. They are specific and numbered.

Every electron in each atom has the exclusive energetic status that is precisely repeated for equally located electrons throughout the atomic world, for this same reason: physical reality has no room for other solutions. And the same applies for protons, neutrons and subparticles. They represent the exhaustion of solutions rendered by an almost inexhaustible rich Universe.

Complexity does not change the specificity of constructions. On the contrary, nuclei acids are precise designs, codes, and clocks, which imply higher control and more coordination. If there were other possible codes, they would have appeared some place on Earth and profusely as the current code does. There is none, as there are no proteins with randomly-linked aminoacids that would have represented the *association by chance*.

To think of the origin of life as common to all species is the logical consequence to see *chance* as the cause of life. As such *chance* is so improbable, there could be only one such miracle and all must depend and generate from it. (Where are the non-miraculous occurrences?) Little thought has been given that to produce DNA-code by *chance* entails admitting that *chance* has performed an unended list of miracles: aminoacids, proteins, nucleotides, membranes, cells and man…with the same dice. Which, by the way, may be about every theory of Physics.

I share in the blame for misleading the reader when shouting: *evolutionary invention!* to stress a few critical points. There are no inventions falling spectacularly in the middle of normality. The normality is made up of myriads of inventions sparkling at every micromillionth of a second and all subjected to the harmony of physical reality. When could lawless *chance* have squeezed itself in the Creation?

The evolutionary evolvement of the DNA-code was systematic, regulated and depending on preceding surrounding structures. It was *gradual,* extensive and *largely general* because no matter what was the evolutive strand that mothered a creature, the molecular realities do not have many other alternatives.

The *type of coding* belongs to *the nature of matter-energy* while the *encoded message* does not. The coding language is essential to the system of life, while the encoded message is essential to the *individual species*, but accidental to the general system of life.

Recapitulation.- The evolvement of nuclei acids, with all probability, has been initiated in *tremendous amounts* in the seas. The different rates of evolution and encoding messages mark the distinction among creatures. There is only a quasi-universal code because this limitation is forced by the nature of reality. The doctrine of the common origin results from the mix-up between the essential and the accidental, which I hope to clarify further along the course of this thesis establishing the universal essences that govern the evolution and systems.

CHAPTER VIII. – LIMITATION OF KNOWLEDGE COMPATIBLE WITH THE THEORY OF SYSTEMS.

Opposition to the proposition that matter-energy freely decide upon the meaning it draws from information will never be substantiated for the whereabouts of the microworld are experimentally accessible only up to a limit. Almost a century ago it was determined that concrete reality cannot be known beyond a certain point. Every physical reality had erected a privacy-like zone, an inscrutable domain banned to any other reality. That territory not only evades inspection now but will also evade inspection forever. The most sophisticated devices or those yet to be devised will be unable to examine or to investigate the innermost core of matter-energy because measurement is not possible. Not because the inadequacy of technology but rather because the very nature of the quantized universe.

This transcendental principle -as previously explained- was enunciated by Heisenberg and it is mathematically expressed by the *uncertainty relations* $\Delta M \times \Delta V \geq h$ where ΔM is the *uncertainty* of the momentum or impulse of the element in question (impulse = mass x speed) and ΔV is the *uncertainty* of its position, **h** being the quantum of action, the smaller amount of action ever found, that is $6.626 \cdot 10^{-24}$erg.sec (action or power = energy x time).

The physical meaning of this is that we shall never be able to establish simultaneously the position of a moving object and its momentum with total accuracy. The product $\Delta M \times \Delta V$ may have values equal or multiples of **h**, but not less (or a fraction of them), as the elemental quantum of action is an unbreakable unit given the quantized character of matter-energy. A smaller value would indicate a fraction of the final unit **h**, and that is theoretically impossible.

Thus, the more precisely the position of a movil is given, the less accurate would be the measurement of its momentum regardless of the efficiency or capabilities of the instrumentation. That encompasses the capabilities of improved or novel future technologies.

The same *relation of uncertainty* binds energy and time

$\Delta E \times \Delta t \geq h$. The product $\Delta E \times \Delta t$ has also the dimensions of action. Here Δt is interpreted as the life of a state and **ΔE** the energy associates to such state. In a state of a very short life the *uncertainty* of measuring the energy of that particular state increases. When the state's life is close to zero, the energetic *uncertainty* grows to infinitum and **ΔE** cannot be assessed.

Consequently, it is also not possible to know simultaneously the kinetic and the potential energy of subatomic particles for the reason that the former, which is E_k = momentum^2 **x** mass, is related to the *momentum*, and the later – potential energy- is dependent on its *position* with respect to the other particles. The Heisenberg's equation tells us that to give value to both –momentum and position- simultaneously and with accuracy is not possible.

Take for instance one electron. The most that can be said about it is that it appears to us *housed in a cloud of probability* each point defining the probability to be the electron in such spot. For, if we pinpoint its exact position, then, the *uncertainty* about its impulse would be infinite.

Furthermore, the Quantum Theory explains that observation or instrumental detection introduces changes in the *observer* and in the *observed,* and that makes it impossible in theory, and therefore in practice, to *know* the independent reality of things and/or to reach the ultimate causes of phenomena. These statements of the Quantum Theory are totally compatible with the basic notion of the theory of systems **"that it is impossible to reach the *meanings* that physical reality draw from information or to detect the *pre-acting energy or freedom* of elemental particles."**

The self-imposed limitations of the Quantum Theory do not end here. In addition, it contends that "the *improbable* exists in the realm of the *possible* and could materialize in rare instances." This admission is of paramount importance to this thesis because it clearly states that "the *exception to the law* is *possible"* and *that* is precisely the crucial proof of the existence of freedom of decision: freedom to escape the dictates of general law, freedom to defy general behavior and order either *pre-established or superior.*

(In the last few years there have been attempts to modify the Quantum Theory towards more individualistic predictions by the so call Hidden Variable Theories. Such studies are in the preliminary phase of determining if the mere existence of these theories is compatible with the quantum principles. Apparently there is not, thus, tilting the balance in support of the theory of systems. This subject lies beyond the scope of this book.)

The point is that current physics does not and cannot offer clear-cut information about the essential world of the ultimate elemental realities. It speculates about their behavior, rating the speculations in the mathematical wave functions that treats subatomic particles as *probabilities or tendencies to exist* rather than concrete factual realities. When one event is observed or measured, the case is stated in these or similar terms:

"One of the *possibilities* of the wave function has collapsed into a tridimensional observable *event*, while the rest of the *possibilities or tendencies* had vanished." Thus, it equalizes the **real**, the concrete, with the **conceptual probability** described by the wave equation. How did the collapse of the wave happen? And, what agency caused it? The answers to these questions are left to **chance**, a disguised substitute for "no answer".

In addition, the intimate intelligence and freedom of elemental particles cannot be detected for another fundamental reason which is, that they are *abstract* faculties and as such more elusive than the *concrete* reality that houses them already established to be unreachable. Rather, the physicist should turn to the hard evidence of the presence of intelligence and freedom in biosystems, and ask himself: When or by what process did freedom and intelligence spring in the biosystem world? Are these not the most debated issues of all times and the proper field of the physicist? Overwhelming contributions to the subject from each corner of our culture pour in torrents. For everyone's hat hangs upon the solution of this enigma, the religious, the philosopher, the jurist, the rebel, their common denominator standing that freedom and intelligence are here in the universe in one form or another.

Ironically, extreme empiricists do not embark on the debate despite *physical reality* being their proper field of exploration, never mind how they dissect *concrete* reality. They stick to experimental data and blinding themselves in such a narrow frame they attribute the cause of phenomena, (not mention made of human decisions), to a myth, a mental construct: **chance.** The bridge from myth, to habituation, to addition, is insensibly crossed to sink in lack of thought flexibility. The result is a loss of receptivity to understand physical reality, and consequently to reject this *unreal*, *virtual* tool schemed by the mind. Thus, *intelligent* and *free* men sternly ignore or deny these same faculties of intelligence and freedom to the rest of the universe despite its proven ability to evolve progressive *orders* without human help or human comprehension of said orders.

Where in the road of evolution is the bridge, or the quantum jump, between free-intelligent systems and non-free, non-intelligent ones? Uncomfortable as it is for science, it still remains unresolved the duality of body and soul, of life and inanimation, of man's intelligence and control **popping out** from a universe whose *components* are *incapable of processing information or making decisions of any degree,* as modern physics alleges.

The above referred are but a few of the inconsistencies and unsubstantiated principles sailing nowhere if biosystems' intelligence and freedoms are not incorporated into scientific inquire.

What lies beyond the impenetrable barrier of experimental reality? Are *the imponderable* open to the human mind?

CAUSES OF ACTION: AUTONOMOUS, IMPOSED AND SUBORDINATED WILL.

Let's talk about the energy at play in the following situations.

1. – A man is inside of a box that has a door open to the outside. Excepting any other circumstances, we shall agree that he is free to stay inside or to leave the box, and sooner or later he will go out. The energy he uses to move is his own energy; his actions are free only depending on the decision of his autonomous *will.*

2.- In a second situation the door closes with the man inside and the box is being forcefully shaken in various directions. He helplessly swings at the rhythm marked by the box, like a ball in Brazilian maracas. The shaking energy is external to the man. Now the man has lost his freedom of movement because his moves respond to the effects of an external *will* imposed upon him.

3.- The biosystem man in either situation still seems able to control other actions like living functions, molecular reactions, activity of his electrons, etc.., upon which the shaking energy is not specifically directed. Obviously the components of his body are subordinated to the *whole system* for they will behave differently out of the system. If a few cells are extracted and transferred to a plate of nutrients, they would grow wildly and reproduce following a *will* of their own whereas in the body their *wills* bend to the discipline established in the organization. Those components possess a *will* of their own and the *integral will* of the biosystem is not blindly or coercively imposed upon them.

The earthworm will serve to illustrate to us these controls. This creature when dissected in several pieces each of them becomes a new worm with a *will* independent of that of the mother-worm and of the *wills* of the other newly produced worms. These *wills* are not new creations but new expressions of the same *wills* that before the partition were subordinated to the *whole,* to the *autonomous will* of the worm.

Energetic interrelations within a system radically differ from alien impositions that obliterate them. The integral and subordinated *wills* -on one same system- are related by genesis, structure and purpose evolved for the interest of the *whole* and upon the interests of the members. Thus, *wills* are implicit voluntary accords; the integral *will* reflecting and containing the internal *wills* of every component.

From our point of view, three types of actions are going on in our box game: **free, imposed** and **subordinated.**

Free and *subordinated actions* are *willed* by the system and its components, and work for its well being because the system's intelligence has an appreciation of its own good, that is the *meaning* it derives from information. These actions are conductive to order, organization, and evolution. In the cases of *imposed action,* because these are not guided by the systems' intelligence, its well being is ignored, not felt, nor cared for. These actions tend to equalize, to level. They are the ones that cause destruction of orders and organizations, that abort systems' growth and evolvement impeding creation. In total ignorance, *imposed wills* render unsuccessful the *meanings* upon which self-organization is erected, and therefore make ineffective the systems' reception of information.

The box insider represents any system of the universe.

CHANCE AS CAUSE OF ACTION.

Modern Quantum Theories eradicate the connections of causality predicted by the Classic Physics. Under old principles future physical conditions can be predicted by knowing the initial ones. For instance, given the speed, time and direction of a mobile, its final point of arrival can be predicted. However, not any more under the current views for this determinism implies the idea of *continuity* and *causality* among physical realities that has no place where matter-energy appears in discrete indivisible quanta. If quanta are separated, they cannot be the cause of phenomena! The Quantum Physics are probabilistic, descriptive, leaving the cause of phenomena to **chance**, blind, irrational **chance** absent of past and future —as we conceived it— while totally negating any role, drives or purposes to the playing elements: the quanta. That is, physics leaves the managing of the universe in the hands of pure *instant lottery* since the beginning to the end leaving concrete reality reduced to mere indistinguishable chips.

Let's go to the mathematics of such a position. The laws of **chance** are expressed by the *calculus of probabilities*, a mathematical tool that works *only* in absolute disorder. Its results are valid when obtained in situations where disorder is total. Therefore, should the universe have a slight symmetry, orientation, order or pattern, the laws of **chance** will not apply to it. And it happens that the universe, since it is in operation, never was in perfect disorder, and at present, universal order is undeniable, appalling, permeating all space, astounding in all systems, continuously evolving and regulating physical realities and new orders. An awkward burden for **chance** to carry when it can only govern disorder!

In addition, **chance** produces disorder out of order. Somebody properly said that **chance** is "the daughter of disorder as well as its morher". **Chance** is born from disorder and is the generator of it! Fairly consistent with this premise, the physical laws tell us that the universe *tends* and will *end* in absolute disorder at a maximum of entropy (entropy is a measure of disorder), and is running toward this end...irreversibly. We must agree if **chance** is the sole agency of universal operation and never to be substituted by any other cause of action.

Physics thus explains that, from the initial chaos after the Big Bang, *orders* evolved...by **chance**. How come, we may ask, when the first *order* made its entrance in the creation, it was not crashed into disorder by the same agent – **chance** - that eventually will return *all orders* to final disorder? Was **chance** paralyzed -so to speak- during the evolution of the innumerable *orders* of the Creation? Or was it progressively inactivated with the accelerated production of them? And as the number of **orders** is incredible great so is the number of unanswered questions posed by declaring **chance** to be the quantum cause of action.

Now let's abandon the grandiose picture of the Creation and see how **chance** applies to local occurrences, a humbler scope in which **chance** might be justified to be the cause of action. First of all, to claim that **chance** is the cause of action, *disorder* must be verified in the specific circumstances of the event in question and in the physical realities to be considered. Now, *isolation* from any influential *order* is absolutely needed to secure local disorder. That refers to internal and external *orders*. Here we already run into problems. Internal *order* is unavoidable. I do not know of any physical reality in *total disorder* and/or immune to any influence. Gravitational forces permeate the universe. In fact, Professor Bell demonstrated mathematically -in 1964- that *local isolation* and the *statistical predictions* of Quantum Mechanics are incompatible. One of such predicaments shall be false. **If** the *predictions* are right, *isolation* is not possible and the laws of **chance** do not apply. **If** *isolation* is possible, then the *quantum predictions* are not. Thus, the very existence of **chance** in restricted areas hosting matter-energy or systems is a theoretical impossibility.

193

After this preamble it does not come as a surprise the fact that *probability schemes* fail to explain any order and structure, and that the attempts to reason the origin of life by **chance** had been abandoned on the spot without further development. Some incipient efforts rather to discourage said adventure come to my mind. As early as half a century ago Professor Charles Eugene Guye calculated the volume of substance necessary to make a protein of molecular weight = 2,000 (2000 times the weight of the H nucleus)...by **chance**. It should be approximately a sphere of *elemental materials* with radius 10^{82} light years long. The radius of the universe is of the order of 10^{10} light years. That is, **chance** needs about 10^{72} universes **full** of raw materials -our universe is for the most part empty- to make such protein, whose weight, incidentally, is less than the simplest one in the human body. Wisely the professor made quite a number of simplifications in arriving to this figure to save himself unnecessary sweat. Even if **chance** gathered all the universes needed for supplies, still the collisions among atoms to react should occur and the minimum estimated time for these collisions was 10^{243} billion years. As the life of the universe is 20×10^{9} years, **chance** should have been working on making that protein during a time equivalent to 10^{233} universe's lives *before* the Big Bang (10 followed by 233 zeros...if you can imagine such a figure)...**but** (now comes the trick) *without materials!* because no materials existed before the Creation. Nature works faster...in comparison, although by other agents of action than **chance** as visualized by this theory of systems. Matter-energy has in itself the power and cause of action: its *will* and *intelligence*.

After these calculations nobody has dared to calculate the materials or time needed in the manufacturing of DNA by **chance**. With reason enough Einstein did not adhere to the quantum approach and left the issue at: "God does not play dice".

To believe that the discovery of natural laws is due to scientific sagacity and the actual marvels of Nature – not discoveries but factual creation of things and creatures– are due to irrational **chance** is pure extravagant reasoning, to say the least. No matter how widely spread such scientific conclusions, still, they are eccentric to any type of logic.

Let **chance** be brushed out altogether and forever as **cause** of physical phenomena, and let's ascribe order and organization to a more efficient agent: **Nature** itself in its multiplicity and intelligent free action.

FEW SUMMARIZING REMARKS. *Intransferability of essences.*

There is no justification to object that all reality partakes of the essential attributes of biosystems: *ability to extract meaning from information, freedom to decide their course of action, and social drives.* The impossibility to transmit or transfer *meanings* or *freedom* from a system to another is no more of a wonder than the impossibility to transfer pain or pleasure among creatures. *Essences* opposed to *accidents* are intransferable from one identity to another identity for the reason that they are an intrinsic part of the identity itself. Nevertheless those identities endowed with such *essences,* and correspondent effects, should be able to recognize them on other systems by induction from such effects.

If intelligence and freedom are not transferable from one biosystem to another, hence those essences are not to be transferable either in the inanimate world. But the paramount fact that *order and harmony* are the product of intelligence, freedom and socialization in the bioworld makes these faculties to be obvious, although of a more rudimentary sort, in the less complex *order and harmony* of the inanimate world.

Universality of the essential faculties of matter-energy.

I find no problem in accepting man to be an intelligent and free creature; does anybody? Instead, from a religious point of view, I find insurmountable difficulties in accepting the justice of a Creator that gave man intelligence and freedom (both absolutely needed for effective action and survival) while leaving the rest of His creatures without them, nor way to get them because they are *intransferable*. The scientist may raise the same question from another angle: Is it credible that Mother Nature poured solely in man and animals those attributes *essential* to their existence and evolvement? And in such variety of forms and at such precise unpredicted times as the profusion of life reveals? Has Nature filled the universe with information and transferable data not to be used until the appearance of what we call *life*? This is untenable since *orders and organizations* have been originated everywhere in the universe long before man or beast could produce any of them.

On the other hand, **order** is not a being, an entity springing from a vacuum and imposing itself upon physical inanimate reality. **Order** is a pattern worked out *from and with information*. (Matter-energy and their interrelations are *the information, the transferable,* while their identities and essences are intransferable.)

As **chance** has no qualities to cause or to support *order* there must be an agency in the universe to process information, present in all space at all times, and none **is** in the entire universe other than elemental matter-energy and their emerging systems. Thus, to physical reality, from its most elementary form to the most complex, shall be ascribed the *universal* cause of order, and therefore the *intelligence* and *will* to process information.

Basically evolution is an *informational game* of building pieces upon pieces, orders upon orders since the beginning of time when the only players were elemental matter-energy.

Association implies intelligence and freedom.

The wave aspect of matter-energy, the traveling character of waves, and the limited volume of the universe brings about the irretrievable communion of Nature. A non-intelligent universe unable to work stable relations would have remained a huge container of perpetually colliding materials where no association was ever possible. Association requires *ordering*, *intelligence* to organize information into satisfactory meaningful relations, *time* allotted to the task, and *freedom to decide;* that is, power to select action. Should matter-energy have been incapable to interpret information and/or to decide to enter into stable associations, evolution would have been impossible. It was not the case. Starting with an elemental *meaning and freedom,* association produced a sequence of orders with higher and higher levels of *intelligence* and *freedom* as organization grew.

Intelligent association is fully corroborated by universal reality, systems' properties, and detectable effects of control-energies.

Willed and compelled action in Nature.

The examination of the actions going in our box shows that *willed* action leads to order and self-organization, while *compelled* action tends to disorganize the system upon which it acts. We may say that our universe as a whole is a *willed* universe because even if *compelled* action acts upon an objecting reality, that action is *willed* by another reality or realities with their own *wills.* In other words, in the scenario of *compelled* action we witness a battle of *wills* which generally ends in incorporating the inferior system into a superior one. The act to eat is to transfer molecules from one system to another. It makes sense to evolution. In the eating of an apple its molecules get up-graded, incorporated to the new animal system, and now able to take part in a more complex operation. Crystallization, for example, compels atoms of the solution to join the crystal which is a structure superior than that of the errand atoms in the solution and invest them with capabilities which they had not before. As a result **information** increases and **entropy** decreases.

Entropy is a measure of disorder, disorganization, unpredictability, randomness, lack of control, lawless and related concepts.

Information, on the other side, is a measure of order, organization, structure, predictability and control. In fact the same function that defines *information* with a negative sign is used to define entropy. The one is mathematically the opposite of the other. I am referring to *information* in its broadest meaning. All physical reality **is** information. The Shannon Theory of Communication narrows the concept of *information* to that particular information *considered* in a specific process, structure.., etc, not referring to the total information constituting *natural* reality.

When *spontaneous* associations take place, or a superior system assimilates an inferior one, there is a sharing of information, production of orders, organizations and structures, and the generation of new *control- energies*. By this, *information* increases while *entropy* decreases. Energy up-grades. And because successful associations come about throughout *harmonic relationships*, the measure of *information* is also a measure of *harmony*.

Sometimes in a battle of *wills,* might and does occur, the contrary that the *winner* is a less organized system or systems. This type of phenomena, pushed by external, ignorant, blind *compulsion*, carries the degradation of systems and energy, and the destruction of order and organization. In these cases *information* decreases and *entropy* increases. Such occurrences projected against the background of the universe and evolution are the anomalous. To predicate that *the* **entropy** *of the creation is irreversibly increasing to a maximum that will mark the doom of the universe* (as the quantum theory does) is to stretch anomaly out of its limits.

Spontaneous association is anti-entropic. Evolution is evidence of an intelligent universe where the non-intelligent action and degradation of energy **is** the entropic exception.

It has been estimated that the minimum amount of energy consumed in transmitting a bit of information by entropic processes is 9.56×10^{-24} Joules per bit per $K°$. That means, that with the flow of information going on in the universe by this time all physical reality would have vanished should *entropy* have its way. Instead reality is still here, and the Creation has grown, evolved and multiplied.

SOLUTION TO THE MAXWELL'S PARADOX.

Natural intelligence and synthetic intelligence are processes *essentially* different. Natural intelligence arises from elemental *essential* intelligence and freedom, and *willed* association. Synthetic intelligence **is** *compelled* action, based on chained mechanisms.

There is a sure degradation of energy in the operation of *synthetic* intelligence. This demonstrates the inability of *synthetic* intelligence to produce what *natural* intelligence does: decrease of entropy.

Maxwell devised a mental construct to *create order out of disorder,* which is impossible under the laws of Physic that equates physical reality with synthetic intelligence. It goes as follows. A box filled with molecules at random has a wall that divides the contents of the box in two parts. The wall has a small door and a minuscule demon open and closes it allowing to enter in one portion of the container the swifter molecules. The slower ones remain in the other portion. After awhile an *order* has been established (the most energetic molecules segregated from the others) which signifies an increase of information and a decrease of entropy. This is contrary to the second law of thermodynamics that expresses the necessary degradation of energy in all physical processes.

The paradox was never solved and never will be because in the process the demon's intelligence had been disregarded and *that* is the *fundamental factor* of action. In the universe Maxwell's demon that *creates order out of disorder* is **not** outside of the molecules guiding their traffic. It **is** inside of them. The demon is the *intelligence and freedom* of the molecules, the *intransferable features* that trigger *spontaneous action...* and where this demon **is,** the second law of thermodynamics and increase of entropy certainly do not apply. For this reason they do not also apply to our universe. Thus, the Maxwell paradox that requires its demon to create **order** comes to prove inequivocally that matter-energy has the intelligence to process information and the power to decide action.

UNIVERSAL EVOLUTION.

Science has already proven the spontaneity of the self-organization of matter-energy in innumerable cases. That is, for matter-energy to have the power to produce order, organization and systems. In other words, *new creatures.* Under the theory of systems we may extend the limits of Darwin's theory of evolution and its scope. The limits to reach all physical reality from the Big Bang to our days. The scope includes the

universal power of creation with which matter-energy and resulting systems are endowed.

Our ancestry goes back to the humble photons who long ago initiated the path conductive to the triumphal achievement of the human biosystem. They deserve a long due token of intellectual gratitude in recognizing that: **"Original matter-energy is the real cause of action via its <u>essential</u> faculties to extract meaning from information and to make free decisions and associations".** Their *essences* are their exclusive realm that we can only assess by their effects because such a realm cannot be reached by instrumentation and our limitation of knowledge.

CHAPTER IX. - INFORMATION AND DECISIONS.

Let's assume that our universe is an aggregate of free intelligent decision-makers consequently acting on information. The degree of intelligence may vary from the very elemental to the highest development and correspondingly with its degree of freedom.

Deciders, elements or systems, must deal with two types of actions and decisions: those regarding their internal functioning and those relating to their external surroundings.

Let's examine upon what information external decisions are based.

EXTERNAL DECISIONS.

A complete knowledge of the particulars of a situation seem to be, at first sight, the soundest ground to make a correct decision. That illusion soon fades, in theory and in practice, because it is impossible to be fully informed of all the contingencies involved in one event. There are not only impenetrable barriers to knowledge but also access to information is oddly distributed among mankind.

More limitations yet abound among creatures less privileged than man. To further complicate things, decisions are made *for a purpose* and only a fraction of the situation's information bears real weight on the end aimed. Selection of the information to be considered takes additional time to that of collecting data.

Animals' survival often depends on split-second decisions, and time is a luxury at the price of life. Time is even more precious for elemental particles constantly running at the speed of light. What time do they allot to their decisions? If total gathering of information affecting a decision were feasible, it would still place the decider in the middle of an ocean of data with no opportunity to check it. Real action is much simpler. Creatures go along existing and functioning, and properly so, by snatching signals that they use as guidance to their activities, similar to car drivers responding to lights, road and labels, while screening everything else. Deciding on key-signals is common to man and animals, to organ and cells, to systems in general, be it a star, atom, colony of insects or a human community. We must assume that the same rule governs the elementary world.

For certain types of decisions there is an *informative signal* that far excels in usefulness everything else, and that is: **the result of the decision.** The *actual result* is the perfect integration of the *needed* information. All related variables -knowable and *even* unknowable- and their effects into the decision, are summed up in the *result*, and *timely assessed* which is a plus-factor in the swift ever-changing character of Nature. On the *result,* the shortcomings or errors of the decision are denounced by the deviation of the goal obtained from the one intended, and corrections can be implemented in subsequent decisions. This method of correction by signaling the *results* back to the decider is being widely used in *synthetic intelligence.*

NATURAL INTELLIGENCE AND TESTING.

Voluntary acting usually proceeds in trial-error fashion by identifying the deviation between aim and actual result. We allude to this method when referring to "testing" or "play by ear".

Observe the *gradual* attempts of an animal in search of food, courting or sniffing danger. He is "testing": guessing, acting and checking the *final* results. He relates *what he wants* to *what he gets*, and tries again adjusting his aim. That is, he corrects his performance in view of the *results* obtained.

A biosystem, in a sense, establishes an invisible connection with the object of his want at the time of decision and concentrates his *will* on it. He focuses and activates only in his *integral will*. His subordinated *wills* and connections can be trustfully forgotten for they blindly and without hesitation will enjoin precisely the action decided by the system's *will*. They are implanted to do a correct *subordinated* job, while to achieve the external goal, the biosystem must get *unmistakable* signals upon which to guide its action. Thus, the success of external acting depends on "testing".

Despite his higher faculties, man normally acts in the same manner. To know every detail could be an intellectual delight but impractical to make decisions. These are made on the knowledge of the results, which encompass all the contingencies a decision may stir, and very frequently a great deal of them are unforeseen and unpredictable. To rely on the *result* is the most intelligent way to *act,* because:

a)   Its simplicity. – To *one* single signal – *the result*– is entrusted the success or accuracy of the decision.

b)   Its completeness. – The *result* integrates *all variables* influencing the process including those that might be unknown or unknowable to the decider.

c) Its efficiency. – The *result* is the direct, valid, unadulterated and integral information, *and all that the decider needs to know,* for information not related to the *result* is automatically eliminated from the process.

The "testing method", then, is indeed well fitted to intelligent deciders, and unsurpassed on its merits. Not surprising that man's crucial activities, business, politics, and technologies are regulated by "testing", although there are plenty of alternatives to decide based in theory, precedent, planning, feelings, intuitions., etc. Still *testing of results* is the preferred one when possible for it affords security, less work and less errors.

Testing becomes even more pressing and useful for creatures less intelligent than man. Unable to assimilate considerable amounts of data their options are but fewer. And hence, they are compelled to testing more and more as their intelligences are smaller. Down the evolutionary ladder this need increases because other avenues of knowing or processing information tend to disappear, and in reaching the elemental level we shall presume that *test by collision* remains about the only available way of obtaining information to make meaningful decisions.

FEEDBACK CONTROL.

Let's state that errors are decisions made with deficient information and/or deficient control. One indispensable item to correct an error is *to know it*. That is obvious even for machines.

At times, decisions made under the best auspices do not bring the effects sought because unexpected circumstances influence the main stream of action. Yet, erroneous results are useful in the sense that they serve as signals to correct future attempts.

After a decision is made, the relation between the *actual* occurrence and the *goal* achieved gives *the controller* -man or automatic instrument- clues for the adjustment needed. Today automatic control is routinarily engineered into instrumentation. This type of control based on feeding back the results of an action has been labeled **negative feedback control** or **feedback** for short. Communication engineers originally quoted the term **feedback** in connection with radio operations. The information upon which the correction is done is called *feedback information.*

The reader might have noticed already the similarity between *synthetic* feedback and *natural* testing.

Control through feedback information is well spread to every technology and actually recognized as the normal operation of spontaneous phenomena. Literature in diverse fields uses its own nomenclature in referring to it. Synthetic self-regulation, servomechanisms, close control, close loop, biological reflexes are but a few of them.

Feedback control stepped firmly and consistently into industrial endeavors along the eighteen century, although 2,000 years ago some gadgets with controls based on *feedback principle* were in vogue. In those earlier ages, float regulators were in use to fill tanks of water automatically and with few alterations, those archaic mechanisms have been adopted in modern domestic cisterns. The ball that floats on the water is the *informative* agent. When it reaches a certain level, the engranages attached to it close the valve that controls the entrance of water thus securing the right level.

Industrialization created the need of servomechanisms on grand scale. Several patents were granted to float regulators to check the water levels in boilers of steam machines. The auto-controls of windmills, rarely used in the previous century, proliferated. They were designed to modify the direction of the main wheel of the mill so as to always face the wind. One small wheel was added to the big one forming a right angle with it. The small one did not rotate when it was aligned parallel to the wind, but it rotated when the main wheel changed position and its rotation forced the turning of the main one until it faced against the wind. In this way the mill worked constantly at full effectiveness.

Another class of *feedback* regulators is the thermostat, fashioned to control the source of heat in order to maintain the temperature of an area at certain range.

The field of electronics has made possible an extraordinary variety of *negative feedback* controls. Automatic controls are available to every mechanical or electrical operation from the simple steering devices to the more sophisticated manufacturing operations and chain proceedings. Feedback mechanisms had practically replaced manual labor in every branch of industry.

Until the forties, though, feedback mechanisms were no more than an *art* restricted to technological advances. Theoretical studies were initiated by Norbert Wiener (1948) who was the first to precisely define **feedback control** as "*a method of controlling a system by inserting into it the results of its past performance*". Weiner unambiguously stated that the process of self-regulation (referring to synthetic intelligence) must have two elements: 1) purpose (teleological aspect), and 2) the use of "negative feedback information" (the term *negative* indicates that the information flows in the direction opposite to the process).

Without feedback information no interaction can be worked out between the *actual* output of the system (the real process) and the *aimed* output (the desired result). The difference between both is the *error*.

NATURAL AND SYNTHETIC FEEDBACK.

Weiner went further, proclaiming that **feedback control** is the foundation of every self-regulating system in the world, referring to natural phenomena. Long before Werner, it had been recognized that most physiological functions operated under the *feedback* principle. For instance, the body's responses to external stimuli or stress, sweat mechanisms, and those steadying the body's temperatures, blood pressure and levels of glucose, oxygen, and CO_2 are subject to *feedback* controls.

The implication that *feedback* regulation is common to natural and to synthetic intelligence **in all its aspects** is totally **false**. For this reason it is of extraordinary importance to stop here, to clarify and solidify concepts.

Weiner was right in the analogy of the processes, testing by *natural* intelligence and feedback by *synthetic* ones. But a fundamental error is committed by fusing natural and synthetic intelligence (and their functions) into the same and single class because they are two entities **essentially** different in themselves and in their functioning. Natural intelligence is a **natural reality** no matter how inaccessible. Synthetic intelligence is a **production** of the first. They differ as cause and effect. The engineer **is** intelligent. The computer, car, airplane are **produced** by the engineer's intelligence and work. They have **no** intelligence on their own but the sole intelligence that the engineer imparted to them.

Let's illustrate the matter from another angle.

It has been said that erroneous results are cause by deficient information and/or deficient controls. In dealing with *natural* intelligence there is another cause of error and that is: *free decision*. Very intelligent creatures can and often make erroneous, illogical decisions, even when being adequately informed and having full control of the situation. *Synthetic* intelligence does not run such a peril. Correct information and correct controls are bound to yield correct results in working instruments or machines. Therefore, if the number of errors is taken as an index of intelligence we arrive at the absurdity that *synthetic* intelligence is superior to *natural* intelligence because the later errs, and frequently, while the former does not.

The temptation to believe such absurdity is enticing when comparing an impressive computer with an insignificant virus. The computer easily handles fantastic amounts of information at incredible speed. Undoubtedly the virus will miss the intellectual contest against the computer in all counts. However, *natural* beings **evolve**, and spectacularly so. *Synthetic* products **do not evolve.** Evidently they are two strikingly opposed things, as well as their productions. It is not possible that from equal source types the one inclined to error finds its way to set forth progressing orders and organizations, in short, evolution. And the other -free of errors- does not advance **one iota** towards self improvement, for not mentioning the capability of self-supporting that remains forever naught.

Of those two contestants, the one has **natural intelligence,** the other has **no intelligence** at all, it has **information** (to miss this distinction brings about the paramount confusion prevalent in current terminology). Natural and synthetic intelligence are related to *information* and should be measured by their *content of information* because it is the only measurable dimension on which both can be *assessed*, but the "relation" to it is quite apart. *Synthetic intelligence* <u>is</u> **information** embodied in the gadget whose function is simply *to match information.* **Natural intelligence** instead extracts *meaning* from *information*, and *meanings* are solely related to the *identity* of the natural creature: element or system. *Natural intelligence, meanings* and *identities* are *not transferable. Synthetic intelligence* is *transferable* because it is nothing more than *information*. It is a calculated plan implanted in the machine. The same plan can be implanted in another machine. It is the engineer's idea materialized in a design, in a set-up, in an artifact. The idea imposed upon the materials do not alter the essential faculties of their identities. Their intelligence and freedom to decide remains untouched now and forever, in the machine or out of it. *Ideas* so materialized are transferable, are *information,* while *abstract ideas* and the *meanings* they *might signify for the system, that* is not transferable, *that* is *essential* to that system and to that system exclusively.

Car or computer does not owe its character to the essential faculties of the materials with which it is built, but to the way they are placed together. The *essences* of its materials are not an addition to the computer's design. As such, the computer is a *container of information;* its interrelations are not harmonically evolved but *imposed* by nuts and bolts; its functioning is entropic with degradation of energy eventually ending into rusty materials. The virus on the other hand is *intelligent*; its functioning anti-entropic; its interrelations self-produced and harmonic rendering creation upon creation.

The flow of entropy definitely marks the distinction between the *natural* and the *compelled* action and so does the feedback operation. *Natural* testing or natural feedback is *anti-entropic* while *synthetic* feedback is *entropic*. From now on I will refer to both as **feedback** in general.

AN INDIVIDUALISTC UNIVERSE.

By the said I hope to have persuaded the reader, if he/she is of the opposite persuasion, that the engineer can only transfer what we familiarly call *concrete ideas* but not his *intelligence and abstract ideas*, nor the meaning and feelings that such ideas arouse in him. This pronouncement is tremendously basic, for such is **the universal character of natural reality, its intransferable essences.** In other words, no intelligence of a natural system can be transferred to operate another natural system. Intelligence and freedom are exclusive to every system, they evolved by the interrelations within *that* system. They are in the *essential province of its identity*. It is the case that systems *within* another system, as cells in a body, or DNA in the cell, still preserve the absolute privacy of their essential faculties. You shall test your own body. It will convince you that your intellect —as superb as it is— does not know anything of what your liver, kidneys or DNAs may know or may decide. These govern their realms in their most comfortable secrecy. We perceive their output of *information and action* as humans communicate by language, but the innermost *meanings* are concealed by impenetrable isolation. Researchers James Watson and Francis Crick figured out how DNA is made up but nobody can built a model of DNA's intelligence and freedom of decision. These are abstractions that defy instrumental reflection.

External information interrelates the universe, which paradoxically is made up of individual entities *in absolute isolation*. Natural action is the *identity's response* to the perception of information based on the *meaning* that such information has for the identity.

Information and essences of the identities can be envisioned as the external and the internal counterparts of natural reality, the communicable and non-communicable of physical reality, the body and the soul of the universe. In the context of this theory, freedom and intelligence are indiscriminately distributed, for all reality is filled up with these faculties, up to its own capacity, so to speak.

OPPOSITE DIRECTIONS OF ACTION.

The concept of **entropy** is of great value to this thesis because it postulates the **degradation of the energy** indicating by this that energy dissipates to less useful forms and does that irreversibly in all phenomena. Erroneously this viewpoint has been applied to **all** action, *natural* as well as *artificial or synthetic.*

In any event, this view initiates the concept that energy has a *qualitative* aspect and paves the road to the novel **energy-control** concept. By establishing that entropy runs parallel to *energy degradation,* then, conversely, the decrease of entropy -that comes with the *increased amount of information* in the production of *new orders*- should occur with an *up-grading of energy.*

Physics notion of degradation of energy relates to the *spontaneous* flow of physical energy. Heat spontaneously goes from hot to cold; water runs from high to lower levels. But, what about the *spontaneous* behavior of natural reality, the flow of evolution, the displays of natural control? Something is missing in that *qualitative* appreciation of energy, and that is, the essential faculties of energy: *intelligence and freedom, and the contribution that information makes to such faculties.* This thesis expands the notion of energy to that of **energy-controls** and incorporates *information* to the equation of action.

But let's, at this point, set aside the *abstract essences* of matter-energy, and consider solely the relation between phenomena and information. The immediate formation of *orders* by the enjoining of information, or destruction of such *orders* by decreasing or destroying information, is just the missing link in a more inclusive and complete notion of up-grading or downgrading energy.

A process or action leads either to an *increase of information* or to an *increase of entropy.* Both are mutually exclusive. The following tables illustrate the various effects of actions when taken into account the *information* factor. Class A, processes with information increase, conveys an up-grading of energy and a simultaneous decrease of entropy. The opposite occurs with processes in the second table Class B where entropy increases at the cost of information.

CLASS A.- INFORMATION INCREASE (Up-grading of energy)	CLASS B.- ENTROPY INCREASE (Degrading of energy)
Natural association	Dissociation
Harmony	Disharmony
Control	Loss of control
Order-structure	Disorder
Organization	Disorganization
Evolution	Degradation
Creation	Destruction

Spontaneous processes promoting association or increasing information are **anti-entropic**. They are the ones devised and brought about by natural reality, freely and intelligently. Actually the increase of information in one action results in the increase of all effects listed in CLASS A. **Entropic** processes produce the effects listed in CLASS B. These are compelled by intelligence alien to the compelled system and will degrade irreversibly the energy of the system and of the universe.

A UNIVERSAL CODE OF CONDUCT.

The universe is a system far superior to man and like every other system it is an intelligent one. Its intelligence measured by its content of information is inexhaustible, beyond the imaginable by human standards. Thus, besides being the origin, cradle and support of man, the universe is a teacher from which we may learn to no end. Of its physical activity we know that it is in continuous expansion, evolvement of orders and increasing information. Its universal harmony and stability render credit to its *moral* teachings. Should we ignore its moral code of behavior we will be thrown into the most foolish of wars against the most powerful, implacable enemy, for the awesome power of the universe parallels that of its grandiose intelligence. A harmonic universe will not welcome disharmony at any level, nor at the human level. It will, then, be wise to try to understand the moral precepts of the Creation.

Human control over creatures, things and events is proudly proclaimed and exercised. To judge by the adverse effects man inflicts on the environment and among his kind, the management of such control is not wise, efficient or even legitimate. *Control* of his own body is also fairly deficient and neglected. Anatomy studies were handicapped until recent times with the old prohibition to dissect corpses and the too late discovery of anesthetics. Just a few years ago most of the body functions were considered *involuntary*, that is, *independent* of the system man. If we add to this the belief in the duality of soul and body we will have an idea of our state of ignorance on the manipulation of human resources. No wonder we are plagued with incurable diseases of body and soul.

Might the tables of Class A and Class B tell us something about the legitimacy and morality of our actions? The moral aspect of the universe is mysteriously followed by the animal world. Animals enjoy a contentment and harmony that humans do not, and I attribute that to the fact that they seem to price social lives above their individual ones. Their *actions* in general fall under the category of Class-A where harmony resides. In eating, the superior organization reaches for the inferior one, so matter passes to higher organizations up-grading its status. In-groups or societies, once morphology or strength has manifested the *rank* (intelligence and control-energy of the individuals), this is respected in its face. Responsibilities and duties are kept without struggle. The instinct to care for the offspring – feeding, teaching, defending- is inexplicable in terms of individual wellbeing and survival. It is clear, though, in terms of the inductive direction of the whole universe to which the creature is connected by infinite strings, past, present and even future. These actions are guided by a social faith, leading to immediate creation and happiness and to an unknown glorious destiny in the long term.

We may say that processes of Class A are *moral* as they follow the direction laid down by the universe at large, in the language of creation, increase of information, decrease of entropy, and evolution. Processes of Class B (if not combined with another of Class A that overcompensate the inevitable dissipation of energy and increase of **entropy** that compelled action carries) would be abuses of the universe with depletion of resources that would result in individual dissatisfaction, social unrest and destruction.

The Tables apply to molecule, cell, body or society, to the physical and the psychic, to the individual as to the local or worldwide extended societies, to the universe itself, because they are grounded indiscriminatorily in the **essences** of physical reality. They might be taken as a **universal moral code** based on scientific grounds, a pragmatic guide that dictates harmony at the base of each enterprise and not limited to specific systems or actions. Good behavior is an immediate human responsibility towards the universe and its creatures, and checking our actions against this **code**, that is in accord with our natural essences, will unequivocally satisfy needs and valid desires, reason and religious beliefs.

CHAPTER X. - INTERNAL CONTROL.

When creatures aim towards external goals, their attention is sharpened and focused on getting information that leads to that purpose. Internal actions do not require this deliberate effort. Systems govern themselves automatically regardless of *the independence of their subordinated wills,* which are aptly adapted. The mere act of eating -if one ponders it- gives an indication of the intelligence of biosystems' mechanisms. It took Mother Earth billions of years of evolution to elevate vegetable orders to the level of animal organization, but now animals assimilate and convert them in their own bodies in a matter of a few hours. And they do it unconcerned with complete trust in the effectiveness of their bodies' mechanisms and the precise coordination of their functions however complex that may be.

To all appearances the internal functions are under so dependable controls that no planing, warning, or precautions are to be added to the decision of the *integral will* for compliance. Man and creature plunge into action, and while concentrating on the external, they totally disregard their internal doings.

The reader may see in this almost perfect functioning a signal of deterministic behavior, that body mechanisms are rigidly chained reactions as those in synthetic intelligence, and that for such reason no errors or deviations therefore happen. Nothing could be further from the truth. Errors and even rebellion of the body's components certainly occur. Nature's laws are general, not absolute. The correct interpretation is that the *integral will* represents the *wills* of all elements of the body and of all their associations. The whole edifice of energies is made up of free consenting energies, and *elementary* activity being close to the speed of light, presumably renews such agreements at every fraction of a second.

The system's organization evokes the arches and aqueducts cemented by the shape and weight of their own stones, each finding suitable accommodation with no binding material in between. Perhaps animals' appeasableness is but a reflection of the accords reigning in their organisms.

The contrast between internal and external actions is striking for obvious reasons. On *internal* action, the information and the control energies are **in** the system, in running operation, coordinated in a general harmony, and joined in the integral and ultimate **will**, the *voluntary will* of the system. The internal mandates are easier tasks than the external ones. Information is not to be sought. Control is not to be conquered for it is established into the system in a peaceful situation contrary to the war that shall be waged against an external *will*. The system is a paradise carefully cultivated by past evolution, ready to harvest at the slight indication of the **will**, while the external world is the *new,* the *challenge*, the *uncontrolled* and likely *resistant,* requiring inventive and venturous action.

Nevertheless, internal acts, at times, as in the case of cancer, defy internal control or so it appears to be the case. Causes and correction of such misbehavior have not yet been determined. In order to ascertain both I shall explore how internal controls might be coordinated in hierarchic structures that develop and replace the centralized operation described in the model of Chapter III.

HIERARCHIC STRUCTURE.

Let's work with a man-made structure: a corporation. The founder of it, being the originator and planner of the enterprise, has access to all data at its earlier stages. Later, the growth of business forces a continual reorganization and while the strings of the corporate net multiply, the hands holding ownership and direction remain the initial two, those of the founder. To keep control under a single command in the face of complexity would require transforming centralized operation and direct supervision into a hierarchic form of management. Labor would split in specialized sections with consolidated inside ties, and from now on the president's decisions would rely on information served to him by the directors of each segregated section.

Hierarchic organization, both in natural and in man-made systems, is an unavoidable advent when centralization becomes impossible, impractical or ineffective. Natural visual examples are the spatial hierarchic arrangement of leaves on trees. Their exuberant foliage is feasible because hierarchic orders take over, otherwise proliferation would produce congestion, inaccessibility to nutrients and decay by starvation. Richness forces the *redesigning* of structure. The tree trunk provides main support and flow of nutrients and it divides into branches whose diameters wisely shrink to conduct smaller and smaller quantities of sap to broader areas of distribution and overall satisfaction.

The word *redesigning* does not reflect the organizing process of Nature. The president of the corporation is the one who re-organizes and *redesigns* his business when congested. The natural system does **no** such *redesigning*! Nature goes ahead along hierarchic structuration *before* congestion arises. And does so without previous blue prints, guided by a most prodigious and expedient prophetic vision, for the hierarchic plan evolved **is** the best of all possible ones in terms of simplicity and efficiency. That is really amazing if we ponder that the hierarchic structuration affects form and function of a very complicated biological affair and that such planning is taking place at an incredible speed. The president of the corporation cannot dream of matching such a feat.

NUMBER OF INTERRELATIONS IN A SYSTEM.

Previously I arrived at a working formula for the number of interrelations in a system. At that time the model was used to visualize the evolvement of energy-controls. Allowing approximations and simplifications, the formula reads:

$$X = \log_2 N$$
$$\mathbf{N} = \sum_{X=1}^{N} 2\left(N/2\right)^N \text{ where } N = 2^x \qquad (1)$$

Where **N** is the number of interrelations in an imaginary system of N elements. X stands for the Class of bonds. Class-1 are bonds of two elements. Class-2 are bonds between two previous bonds of Class-1. Class-3 are bonds between two previous Class-2 bonds, and so on.

Every Class of bonds has a content of information = 2^x. The process of bonding ends with the formation of the last bonds carrying $N=2^x$ bits of information which is information from each and all elements and the same in all the last bonds.

We are already familiar with the potencies of **10** to represent huge numbers in a very easy and simplified manner, but also with equal ease a slight change in the exponent of 10 can transport us from our real dimensions to the most fantastic ones, completely unreal or totally impossible. Suppose that the mass of the Sun is 2×10^{33} gr. By simply writing 2×10^{34} gr. we have the mass of approximately ten suns. If the age of the universe is 2×10^{10} years, just 2×10^{11} years expresses about ten times the life of the universe; 2×10^{12} years about hundred times the life of the universe; 2×10^{13} years about thousand times the life of our universe. And, if the Creation contains 10^9 galaxies, a little variation to 10^{10} galaxies describes **TEN** Creations.

In the formula of interrelations we stumble upon one of these *exponential* functions 2^x (A function is called *exponential* when the variable is the exponent) that although in appearance is innocuous, it **is** insidiously red dangerous. A few digits added to the X of the simple 2^x number and the function jumps to exorbitant and unimaginable values. A tale will illustrate which of these values are compatible with the Earth's dimensions.

Far back in the ages, a King of Persia or China was deceived and embarrassed by the unfriendly 2^x formula. History tells that the inventor of chess pleased his majesty so much with the new chess game that he was granted any payment he would ask for. Loyal to his mathematical inclinations the subject requested one grain of rice for the first square of the chessboard, two for the second, four for the third, and successively doubling the number of grains at each square. Just 2^x grains of rice for each square, x indicating the site of the square.

What appears to be an insignificant request turned out to be an unreachable price. All the rice of the kingdom did not suffice to meet the amount of rice to be placed *in the 32nd square.* The following square, the 33rd, was worth the rice of several kingdoms. Thereafter entire kingdoms were at stake, and multiplying at the same rate of single grains in the initial squares. Solely the last square 2^{64} grains amount to more rice than the Earth can yield. (You may check the figures by weighting a few grains of rice, expressing the weight in potencies of 2 gr. and adding units to the x exponent of 2^x gr.).

Be sure that the formula (1) has a few surprises awaiting you. In it, the 2^x function is more troublesome than that of the chess because x is not the exponent. THE WHOLE $\underline{2^x}$ IS THE EXPONENT of the base N/2. Instead of the exponent being a series of consecutive numbers 1, 2, 3.., etc, the exponent is now *the sequence of grains in the squares of the chessboard* given by 2^x. And instead of 2 being the repeated factor, the base in the exponential formula, the factor now is N/2, N being the number of elements of the system, which is astronomical in the simplest of biosystems. It boggles the mind to guess *the number of elemental particles our bodies have* and *this* is *the first grain of rice* in the new game given by the formula (1).

The chessboard could not carry the rice demanded by 2^x, less can be expected that any system whatsoever could carry the far more exorbitant number of interrelations given by formula (1). Even if the impossible materialized, the interrelations would be overlapping, engulfed in extreme densities; the information conveyed by them would be indiscernible; *meaning* impossible.

Systems should solve the problem of overcrowded relationships without sacrificing internal control. They do so by hierarchic patterning endowed with competent consolidated energy-controls.

Assuming that the Big Bang was the birth of the universe, hierarchic structuration got its start immediately after it, because no matter how small the energy of each interrelation among elemental particles was, the incredible number of them -according to formula (1)- could not coexist at any time in the physical dimensions. In addition, such relations entitled more energy than all the mass of the universe could provide.(See Chapter III). Thus, the Big Bang was almost simultaneous to a collapse into segregated orders of galaxies that for identical reasons subdivided into astro-bodies reducing the number of interrelations to an affordable figure. This is the way Nature routinarily works in *redesigning* hierarchic structures. (The next point elaborates on the effect of subdivision in reducing the number of interrelations of the system.). By this method the Universe still controls its own structure and presumably exerts external control judging from its continuous expansion.

Should social relations not have been *essential* to matter, equilibrium would not have been established by that time. Incipient gravitational forces, or field forces as viewed by Einstein, seem to be *immanent*, and

233

due to them matter concentrated further and faster with the shortening of the distances.

The stars that were being created found themselves driving on the same problem of an unaffordable number of energetic relations. Internal collapse into atomic nuclei was the already repetitive process of hierarchic structuration. Subgrouping now consolidates elemental particles into nuclei held by the novel *strong forces.*

Each star developed atomic nuclei according to its size, from H to He on the Sun-size stars, to the rest of the periodic system in the bigger Supernova. *Strong forces* developed when and where the star-system got the cumulative energy to produce them. Elemental particles in the nuclei, by becoming part of the nuclei-systems, became contributors to powers not possessed by themselves in isolation. Such power was greater in bigger stars invested with more powerful energy-controls. And, when the *integral control* of a superstar was *not* up to the job of subduing the internal energies and emerging radioactivity, the superstar would explode giving birth to lesser systems. Its *soul* would depart. Death in the celestial process as well as in all systems is *the loss of integral control.* Hence it appears to be a universal process. The *creation* of systems that up-grades internal energies to a point where *integral control* may not fit the dimensions of the physical universe and subdivision occurs with the consequent loss of the *integral will* or death.

We habitually identify systems by the perception of their *integral control*. Nuclei are defined as *unities* by their unified control and not for the contribution of its components. Should this control collapse, the nucleus would disintegrate or would suffer transmutation and the *unity*, the *identity*, would no longer exist.

Atoms are considered unities because they are *controlled* structures. *No control* amounts to *no structure*. Molecules, crystals, and in general systems, are identifiable by their interrelations -all included up to the *integral control will*- for, at the light speed of energy, no energy can be stopped in the middle of its runnings. Once elements interrelate in a system, they relate up to the apex instantaneously.

Creatures are systems only while they are alive. At death the *integral control,* the *will,* departs and with it their *identities*, despite the fact that many organs and cells continue working under the control of their subgroups-wills. Insect societies and man communities are similarly identifiable by their *ruling controls*, lasting as they do.

SUBDIVISION REDUCES THE NUMBER OF RELATIONS.

In the model of Chapter III maximum liberty in simplifications were taken (it was considered one *single* relation among two elements because less will be *no* relation.., etc) to stress only and substantiate directly and exclusively the new concept **energy-control**. No consideration was paid to whether energetic overcrowding was ever possible. The content of information of energy increases by bonding. The *final bonds,* which are the most numerous, carry information of all the elements. Thus, the informational content is identical in all of them. It is obvious that the system does not need such repetition of information to make proper decisions. Efficiency calls for alternatives.

Let's see the effect of subdivision on the number of interrelations.

By subdividing a group of N elements into subgroups of n_1, n_2, n_3, such that the sum of them equals N, the number of relations, and repetitive information become considerable reduced.

Taking a group of 16 elements and subdividing them into groups of 4, Table No.2 shows that the number of interrelations in the second plan has been reduced.

The number of bonds at every round decreases dramatically by the subdivision, 24 instead of 120 for

Class-1 with 2 informative elements, 60 instead of 7142 for Class-2 with 4 informative elements; 420 instead of 25,486,230 for Class-3 with 8 informative elements, and 87,990 instead of 324,673,957,718,460 for Class-4 with 16 informative elements. A total of 324,673,983,211,446 relations have been eliminated. That number grows astronomically with every successive Class in systems of more that 16 elements.

See that the *integral controls* of subgroups shall incorporate into new systems otherwise the lack of communication among subsystems would make them four independent systems instead of one single integrated one. We will not dwell now on such a problem.

TABLE No. 2.

Number of bonds.

No subdivision		Subdivided on	Partial savings
Elements	16	4 + 4+ 4+ 4 = 16	----
Class-1 Bond	120	6 + 6+ 6+ 6 = 24	120-24 = 96
Class-2 Bonds	7140	15 +15+15+15 = 60	7140-60 = 7080
Class-3 Bonds	25.486.230	105 +105 +105 +105 = 420	2 5 , 4 8 6 , 2 3 0 - 4 2 0 = 25,485,810

Class-4 Partial Savings are =324,673,957,806,450 - 87,990 =   324,673,957,798,460

The sum of the partial savings in said **4 elements system** will give the total number of bonds saved which is equal to 324,673,983,211,446.

Content of information is given by the formula 2^x, x

being the Class of bond. Thus, content of information is $2^0 = 1$ for the elements; $2^1 = 2$ for Class-1 bonds; $2^2 = 4$ for Class-2 bonds; $2^3 = 8$ for Class-3 bonds; and $2^4 = 16$ for Class-4 bonds.

INTRINSIC AND EXTRINSIC RANK.

The term **rank**, commonly used in relation to biosystems, denotes power to subordinate.

The theory of systems, by postulating that energy **is** empowered to decide over itself, as a pail controls its contained water, considers the *intrinsic* energetic **rank** to be rooted in the very own nature of the energy. That is, the *specific level* of control of self-subordination is the first exhibit of **rank**. Internal actions of systems are explained in Chapter III by the model of a net of energy-controls. From the initial energetic elements every bonding combines energies producing more powerful ones on account of *quantity of energy* and *information it contains*. The first energetic bond among two elements (Class-1) **is** a system in itself, with *control* over the two elements (*intrinsic* **rank**). The control is essential and intransferable. Now the Class-1 bond has a social tendency to associate with other energies and it finds adequate partners in another Class-1 bond with equivalent amount of information (*equal rank*) and will bind into Class-2 bonds, and thus successively.

In this way control-energy and **rank** are being created **simultaneously,** and ascending automatically in the system.

New associations and new relations occur -in the formation of systems- when the underlying ones enjoy a stability and permanence that overlives the trials of the new venture. No molecules are possible without stable atoms. No crystal without stable molecules. No edifice can be erected with disintegrating bricks. Instability of components makes the building on new ones grounded on them impossible and so the evolving harmony.

In the building of natural systems the *initial elements* become *subordinated* to a superior control, Class-1 bonds. In the next bindings the *elements' subordination* to more and more powerful controls Class-2 bonds, Class-3 bonds., etc would be reinforced. Hence the association of components in more complex systems guarantees stronger *subordination* of the *initial elements* to the integral control, and therefore more *stability* of those lowest elements. The greatest forces known, the ones binding particles in atomic nuclei and properly named *strong forces* are an illustration of such *stability* that no known force can break.

A paradox though is plain. The elements are always the same and the up grading of their power comes from the orders they form. But while this power increases when the elements are incorporated into superior orders, the *subordination* of such elements to these orders -*that they create*- also increases. And this might appear to be an abrogation of their own individual power.

Based on these reasonings the subordination of human DNA to the human **integral will** must be **unimaginable.** And so it shall be its *stability*, which makes problems such as cancer a puzzle to us. How can DNA misbehave under the prodigious power of the human body?

Conversely, *extrinsic* control, the control an energy may exert upon another *external* one, is not guaranteed by its own nature for they do not share any content of information. It depends on *imposed control* and that control determines **rank** (*extrinsic*). We are familiar with animals' rituals to assert **rank** in their respective societies. At the core of them is an immoderate and defiant display of themselves aimed to intimidate and subordinate others. Frequently an actual battle is the practical way to decide **rank**. *Extrinsic* **rank**, therefore, is not set up within the energy itself; it is set up a posteriori, in view of the final control externally gained.

RANK AND HIERARCHY.

What happens to the **ranks of control** when the hierarchic structuration takes place generating a system of systems?. No hierarchic design should violate **rank-**

levels that are essentially connected to energy and independent of the path of association the energy takes. **Rank** accurately, inflexibly and gradually climbs up by relating **equal-rank** elements, and later, **equal rank** bonds up to the apex. Logic dictates that equality of rank should cross subgroup lines entirely, at any given time, for only this scheme would insure the *equilibrium* of coexistent groups and subsystems. In the limited space of a system, the domination of a weaker subsystem by a stronger one would occur almost instantaneously, because: a) *energetic* processes run at the speed of light, b) external control is a fundamental capability of systems, therefore also of subsystems. Hence, stronger subsystems in the vicinity of weaker ones would exercise control subordinating these to their *wills,* and c) there is no escape from the system.

Experience proves the above mentioned. The contrary, control of a subsystem over another one due to its superior rank, soon would transpire into tangible realities. The dominant subgroup would emerge in preference to others by incorporating them. Did you ever come upon a *living* isolated arm or leg of a creature? There are no such manifestations. Even lower organisms as the earthworm when split, the parts tend to reconstruct their own *whole structure,* not some organs in preference to others or to expand the spliced segments.

Systems of great complexity are extremely sensitive to internal *rank-equilibrium*. Such balance is especially fragile and delicate in *hierarchic-ranks.* For although hierarchic structuration is not the disintegration of a system to minor ones, but a *redesign* of it to a system of systems, still there seems to be a weakening of relations among separated subgroups in favor of their internal strengthening. It is well known that the destruction of a small part of a forest can throw off the entire forest system in a very short time. And following the arguments creatures are more vulnerable than crystals, molecules more than atoms.

The **equilibrium** among *energy-ranks* demands that the *escalating associative process* that creates them should be coupled by another *rank de-escalating process* that would allow communication among **equal-rank** energies from the top of the integral control to the bottom of elemental energy. **Direct** communication between the *integral* control and lowest *energetic levels* or *elements* does not look feasible on account of the qualitative and quantitative disparity of such energies. Communication among *different rank* energies would break the equilibrium of ranks making it possible for a subsystem to overcome another, as said before. From the integral *will,* bonds would progressively disassociate into their components to finally communicate with the lowest energetic elements in their same elemental language and rank-energy.

This thesis entails annexed opportunities to exercise erroneous *free* decisions against the established order but these would also happen over equivalent **ranks** of energies where communication is possible.

HIERARCHIC STRUCTURES AND FEEDBACK.

Hierarchic structure divides system's information among subgroups. Afterwards they do not share the same information at that level, hence their relations become typically **external** ones. Thus, while a system in dealing with the external world is guided by feedback information, its internal activities are guided in two ways: by built-in information in the **energy-controls,** and by feedback information among factions that do not share built-in information. Actually *any external action* is such because the *system-universe* became a *hierarchic structure* shortly after the Big Bang. The loss of guidance by build-in information was and is always replaced in hierarchies by feedback information.

Feedback mechanisms have been studied in biosystems at the cellular, organic and higher physiological levels. Top expression of them are analytical reasoning, judgments and the rest of familiar human activities. They are not fed by internal sources but by external ones: empirical data, library books and inspiration, to cite a few.

Under these guidelines, far away from infallible, we may now speculate, sketch and debate about possible hierarchic structures to unending lengths. The marvel of Nature's dynamics is that while we squeeze our brains in geometrical and mathematical computations to justify the most rudimentary of models, Mother Nature crystallizes hierarchic structures of extraordinary complexity effortlessly, rightly heading to plans of top efficiency, apparently at first trial, and practically free of error. And it is doing all this each second, night and day, winter and summer, changing the universe in a playful manner irreverent to scientific calculations.

We may adduce as explanation that the making of decisions and meanings *may be* done faster than light speed, or *totally out of time dimension*, considering that each act of the trajectory of a photon shall be anticipated by an speedier decision. Nature surely beats us as planners.

In a universe made of *light* there are two alternatives. Either there is a *decider to compel light-action, or light has the ability to make decisions and meaning out of information* faster than light. The theory of systems sets for the second alternative. To assume one decider behind every photon are too many assumptions to be carried on.

FEEDBACK WORKS IN AN INTELLIGENT UNIVERSE.

It was explained in Chapter IX that *feedback information* provides the opportunity for the correction of decisions, assuming that the decider is an *intelligent* one or an *intelligent* mechanism implanted artificially.

Modern Physics envisions matter-energy totally deprived of any inherent intelligence to interpret information. Here are some immediate thoughts and consequences if this erroneous postulate stands:

1) Information as such, that is, *all communicable physical reality* that constitutes the entire universe would be a waste for lack of an intelligent consumer to perceive and assimilate it.

2) *Feedback information* would be of no value in the absence of agencies that use and process information. Abundant illustrations of feedback in the living and non-living world are amply reported in scientific writings. *Intelligences* themselves develop by *learning* through feedback of one sort or another.

3) What intelligent identity operates the feedback mechanisms that we observe everywhere in Nature? Or for what purpose when the immediate

deciders are incapable of understanding the use of them for lack of intelligence?

4)   As the cause of all events is **chance,** which has *no intelligence*, no memory to store information, the errors should be obviously more numerous than the hits and *chance* unable to correct them by *feedback* or by *internal information*. Both out of its capabilities. Errors against the normal order will pile-up exponentially to total **chaos** in no time, as physics accordingly predicts without estimating the date it would occur. This position contemplates a non-purpose, hostile universe opposed to the actual evidence of an *intelligent, harmonious* one. Harmony takes a lot of intelligence to judge for the struggle it takes to reach human harmony alone.

5)   The notion of a non-intelligent universe is rather untenable, moreover with *the present trend to assess biosystems' intelligence in terms of information.* It inescapably would lead to the evaluation of intelligence of **all** concrete physical reality on the *same* basis of information. In other words: There should be **natural intelligence** where there is **natural information.**

6)   The *universality* of the feedback operation makes plain *at every level* of the creation, that intelligence is available to process and to

interpret information. Or at least somebody shall be able to figure out and explain to us how non-intelligent agents could carry out intelligent feedback processes.

7)   Physics should be the front line discipline to judge our universe to be an intelligent one because **its intelligent laws** are precisely the intelligible matter of physics.

FEEDBACK FITS A FREE AND LAWFUL UNIVERSE.

Feedback methodology fits, works, and is needed, in a generally lawful, therefore, *intelligent* and *free* universe.

For one, feedback solely works where consistency of phenomena and predictability can be ascertained: in situations ruled by general law. Without high probability of average events feedback would make no sense as guidance. It would be unreliable, therefore useless.

On the other hand it is needed where *errors* occur – which will happen only in a *free* universe- to prevent disaster. Intelligent elements with no freedom shall never err nor cause others to err. They would be fatally bound to act intelligently and *feedback would not be necessary*. The laws would be *absolute and universal,* instead of *general*. Potential error exists where freedom does and that deviation from the general law appears at any level of action. Thus, indicating that the universe is *free,* and hereby the *reason that feedback is universally needed,* to adjust decisions in view of own and others' errors.

Chance's laws work in *perfect disorder* where prediction is not possible, errors cannot be corrected, and information can never be processed. A *chancy universe* cannot use feedback mechanisms. Obviously, in an ordered creation **chance** is not a **reality**, it is an empty opinion invented to explain another *unreality* : *non-intelligent, non-free action.* No such action is or ever was in the entire universe according to this thesis.

Conversely, *feedback* is a *real* method ingrained in *reality.* It denounces that *action* **uses** the information served back for a more accurate action, that is to say, that action is *intelligent* and has *purpose.*

Feedback mechanisms are not sporadic, odd occurrences. They have been developed from the beginning of time by all physical reality. They adapt complexity and simplicity with equal flexibility. They are torches of action by bringing to the decider the fruits of his trials for gratification, learning and correction, and ultimately to fit its free action with the harmony of the Creation.

FEEDBACK AND SYSTEMS.

For the sole reason that feedback is a universal tool of action it can be soundly predicted that a *gradient of feedback mechanisms* go all along the way of systems activities. In short: hierarchic structure should be mirrored by a correspondent hierarchical structure of feedback regulation.

Every system has an *integral control* crucial to its organization, which biosystems clearly manifest on their *will*s. The theory of systems extends this view to every *subsystem*. They are in control of their operations. Such control qualifies them as **a** system. The qualification reaches the very elemental matter-energy, whose *will*s are essentially free and in control of the element.

Thus, in the case of a **cell** of a multicellular organism, that **cell** is simultaneously:

1) a system with a built-in *will* exercising internal control and having rank-energy,

2) a subsystem of the body of the multicellular organism whose *will* is subordinated to the body's *integral will*, and,

3) a subsystem of the universe having relations with the rest of the Creation and *subordinated* to the *will* of the universe.

CHAPTER XI. - THE CURE OF CANCER.

Cancer had been defined as a group of diseases having in common one feature: the uncontrolled growth and division of cells. Cancer is not specific to certain organs or cells. It could spring everywhere and once the abnormal cellular behavior starts it might spread to unrelated organs or tissues without showing trace of transmission.

Cancer is not contagious as bacterial infection is; that is, it is not a cell invasion. Nor it is hereditary, therefore *it is not communicable in the genetic material*. And if we add that it is not transmitted from one part of the body to another but might appear in unrelated locations, cancer seems to be a dysfunction *not exclusive to the cell* but to the combination **body-cell** of a particular individual.

Because cancer is *not transferable* **in or out** of the body we may say that cancer is rooted in the inherent *essences* of the system. Those intransferable items! It has more to do with *energy*, and *meanings* and *wills of energy* that with empirical information, concrete reality.

What triggers this cellular dysfunction in the system? The crucial trigger of cancer proved to be unreachable, for all cells potentially can undergo change from normal to cancerous under no stimuli at all or under a diversity of stimuli numbered by the thousand that may *not affect other cells.* To these preliminaries, it shall be added that the complexity of cells is extraordinary in structure and function. Some of their basic mechanisms have been deciphered just in the past few decades. The variety of cells is astonishing among creatures' species and between multicellular organisms, which are precisely the *targets* of cancer, *Unicellular beings are not affected by it.* This is a key reason in favor of the argument that cancer is a **system's** dysfunction, whether inducing cellular abnormality or failing to restore it to normality.

In the body community cells exhibit a strong social behavior that permits the coordination of the innumerable living operations. Even in the extreme situation of cells being extracted and placed in experimental cultures, they aggregate into organized fragments of tissues analogous to those from which they proceed. Such social affinity is not present in microorganisms' cells, which grow free as soon as division ends. Cells of higher organizations have a peculiar *social memory*. A dramatic experiment with marine sponges visualizes their capability and specificity of reorganization. When cells from two or more specimen of different color are dislodged by sieving them through a silk cloth and dispersed in a proper medium, the sieved particles reaggrupate into distinct separate sponges of the original colors. *The success of this experiment closely depends on the number of cells.* If they are under a **critical number** apparently they cannot sum the power to reproduce the original patterns. See Critical Number in the development of a system, Chapter III pg.? where it is reasoned that the system becomes into existence when the energy of interrelations is superior to that of its components. At that point the *integral will* of the system controls the system and it is also able to exert external control.

Cancer cells seem to have lost the sense of belonging and social duty characteristic of multicellular beings, not only in the system but also out of it. Within the body they reproduce disordinately invading other tissues, depleting the system of vital resources and antagonizing most activities. Out of the body *disorder* continues to be the norm. They are completely dissociated from the system and confused about what is supposed to be the healthy acting. They are unregulated because the *system's normal regulation* or *the programming of such cells as part of the system* certainly had failed.

Not only we don't have a cure for cancer, but the problem remains undefined, except for the so broad definition above-mentioned which amounts to lack of definition. Causes have not been ascertained other than in terms of statistical data. There is no sound doctrine or theoretical foundation to interpret or explain cancer, and no predictable solution for it.

Present therapies are based on the destruction of cancerous cells -*not in the cure of them*- and in the alleviation of symptoms. Surgery and radiotherapy are nothing else that cut-off of cancer and whatever tissues host it in the hope that *other cells* will not turn cancerous at a later date. This hope is in general unfulfilled, the patient with part of his body amputated, and his immune resources crippled. Chemotherapy disrupt cellular functioning and with it the cell's life. And clinical immunotherapies are conceived and designed to increase the body's defenses expecting that cancer will be recognized *as an intruder* and killed. Thus, both methods are equivalent to more amputations.

These alleged therapies erroneously treat cancer cells as a *threat* to the body while they are indeed *essential part of it* in need to be restored to proper functioning. The result is that no matter how drastic the medical cleaning job, it is ineffective; moreover damaging. Cancer remains and no doctor has figured out **the cure**.

GENETIC IMMUNITY.

The DNA molecule contains encoded in its structure a colossal amount of information believed to be practically all the instructions of cellular life. The totality of cellular DNA constitutes the genetic material which is mostly located in the nucleus of the cell excepting red cells that have no DNA, and the ones that have lost the nuclei in their terminal stages of differentiation: nails, hair.., etc.

DNAs in all cells are identical, for their way to reproduce, *replication*, renders accurate copies of them. Thus, a liver DNA contains the same information of heart, nerve or brain DNA. Yet, it has not been discovered what makes a cell **select** the use of specific instructions in preference to others, by what mechanisms the liver-DNA out of its code **selects** and only dictates to the cell a *liver- cellular-behavior* and no other. The surge of cancer is moreover surprising giving the adaptability of DNA to any circumstances in order to subserve the overall operation of the body. When a liver-cell, for instance, is transplanted to a muscular or conjunctive tissue it blends with its neighboring cells *acting exactly as they do*. That means that in the new location DNA activates a new set of instructions and silence others. What nullified the *active* tendencies and stimulate *dormant* ones when cells relocate within the body or out of it? Location *per se* does not justify the change of behavior. *Space* does not confer special properties. There must be another key of crucial importance to the whole genetic material that explains its adaptability and specialization.

Besides, it is proven that *non-specific* stimuli elicit *specific* cellular response of a wide range of diversity. All cells are under control of the same DNA with the same set of instructions. What do determine the *various types* of reactions to *the same agent*?

More puzzling yet, DNA is capable of self-repair and when engaged in cancerous functioning DNA does not activates those mechanisms to reshape itself and/or reverse abnormal reactions, as it habitually does in other occasions. DNA self-repair is a process equivalent to an immune reaction at the molecular level, I will name it **Genetic Immunity** to distinguish this new immune concept from the familiar one known as **immunity** or **immune defenses** working at the physiological level.

In rare instances remissions of cancer have been reported when medical treatment has been discontinued or never applied. Cancerous cells already embodied in the patient have been restored to health spontaneously. Consequently with the notion that DNA regulates the cell's activities and no the other way around, these spontaneous remissions shall be attributed to a right response of the DNAs, of the **Genetic Immunity**. They prove that *DNA knows how and does cure cancer*, and so does every other cellular disease for all respond to DNA's regulation. DNA is the repository library of genetic information. The two way street, from health to cancer and from cancer to health, is the familiar province of DNA's intelligence.

Genetic Immunity stands to reason for it is no less that an *essential device of self-preservation* of the *living orders.* From the postulates of this thesis this essential devise derives from the control that **every order or system** (that is, all physical reality that comes into being) **has of its functioning and existence, which entails control of self-preservation.** It is a *universal principle* that shall manifest itself in every living system in a great variety of immune defenses. It is an extension of universal inertia and we may call it in this particular case *bioinertia.* Thus, the commonly named *physiological immune defenses* are but macro scale manifestations resulting from a more elemental immunological phenomenon that has its origin in the DNA, and beyond it, in the most elemental components of reality.

In the hierarchic structure of biosystems they can be found appropriate immune defenses at the elemental, local, organic or whatever physiological level for all living orders need them and quite unexpectedly. Such immune reactions are in fact *biofeedback mechanisms of self survival.*

Genetic immune defenses have been known to rightly operate in rejecting cancerous tissues implanted in healthy volunteers. Experiments conducted in the Sloan Kettering Institute in 1956 report that following a vigorous inflammatory reaction, the cancerous implants promptly disappeared. That is, the genetic immune defenses of healthy people *worked* in the extreme situation of *implanted* cancer to eject it. Most certainly they should reject all carcinogenic agents that are *not* so drastic and consummated stimuli as cancer itself and that have *not* been forcefully *implanted* in the body. The fear to carcinogenic agents is then in most part overestimated.

Given the above premises, the innumerable questions posed by cancer can be reduced to two: What inhibitory agent paralyzes **genetic immunity** in the cure and in the prevention of cancer? Why are the *familiar physiological immune defenses* inactive or ineffective in the battle against carcinogenic agents and cancer producing viruses (or AIDS) that are foreign threats to the body?[1]

The second question was practically answered by Dr. P. Vogt experiments in 1978 (University of California). He discovered that **healthy DNA** can provide segments of healthy DNA to invading viruses to star a tumor. Without these segments the virus does not produce cancer. The intercommunication virus-DNA is not surprising for viruses are DNA's molecules and *the coding of life is the same for all living forms, the same language.* What is surprising is that DNA acts in favor of the *foreign* system, the virus, instead of repelling it as a proper immune defense should do for its system: the body. And here it is the answer: *the immune reaction has obviously failed at the genetic level, where defenses should be initiated and harmoniously related to the rest of the body's defenses.* **Genetic immunity** is defective or wrongly programmed on the DNA.

It is possible that if a tumor grows out of proportion, broad *physiological immune defenses* may get stimulated by the deformity and will destroy it, just as surgery will do, without this action being any proof that the *genetic immune system* is in working conditions. It is obviously not when the tumor was produced. Cancer cells should have been corrected and well behavior restored long before the declared aberration of cancer came about **if** DNA was in good working condition.

AIDS is a clear example of genetic immune deficiency for the fight against the virus should have been carried out (as in cancer) at the DNA level.

ENERGETIC INTERPRETATION.

The difficulties in explaining biological problems arise because the faulty methodology we are used to employ. Genetic, cellular or any physiological action is interpreted as a physic-chemical *wired-in process* consistent with the **concrete** description of phenomena offered by present physics. This conception does not reflects the nature of elemental matter-energy neither the rest of physical reality. In biosystems actual events are initiated always at the elemental level (of matter-energy) before they reach the global expression of detectable occurrences. These are the results of a non-stopping energetic microworld in whose *control* are the palpable, concrete physical realities.

The theory of systems interprets the spectrum of diseases cancer, AIDS, and genetic dysfunctions as disorders of the pattern of control-energies that can be induced to proper functioning by the system itself. That opens a new field, **Clinical Biofeedback at the genetic level.**

CELLULAR ACTIVITY AND CONTROL.

The whole network of the system's energy is accountable for the control of cell's activities including differentiation and dysfunction. The *energetic dimension* commands action on *material reality,* it works faster than cellular wired-in processes due to its light-speed. Thus, the body functions under an *organic energetic control* rather than *wired-in controls of physic-chemical reactions.* The wired-in interpretation of cells' functioning conflicts with the phenomenon of *cellular differentiation,* which is not a sequence of reactions more or less coordinated or even simultaneous, but the formation of a *pattern, at once,* with no intermediate precedents.

Subordinate control in the net of interrelations is exerted from the above, from what it is energetically superior containing more information than the below levels of energy. The development of an organism involves a vast number of DNA *identical* replications and generations of cells by division of each into *two equal ones.* This mechanism does not entail the future construction of a mature creature where cells have acquired peculiar characteristics, diverse organs emerged, and functions complexity overpasses by far DNA and cellular activities. The building of a creature demands more complex mechanisms of evolvement.

Cells of highly organized biosystems contain and manage the information and program of *cellular activity,* and only that. Period! They don't understand organs' functions such as that of the liver or brain, or systems functions such as that of muscular and nervous system or physiological immune defenses.

To discuss the present topic of control of cellular behavior I will tentatively adopt the almost unanimous consensus that cellular activity is mainly regulated by the DNAs. The cell dances -I may translate- to the tune that DNA pleases to play out of its encoded repertoire. Thus, we retain DNA responsible for the normal and the cancerous behavior of cells as well as for the variety of roles that cellular differentiation assigns to each cell. Now with this approach, the enquiry of cellular functions will exclusively focus on the DNAs. Cell activities are to be regarded as subordinated and depending on DNA whatever the modus operandi could be, wired-in processes or energetic control.

Each generation of cells forms a unique pattern of DNAs in the life of the creature and such pattern also changes at each fraction of second considering that the reactions of the DNA are about one million to one hundred million per second. **If** all DNAs are exactly equal because the accurate mechanism of replication,

- <u>what</u> determines the set of instructions to be used in generating the multimillion differences among cells?
- <u>when</u> do DNAs start cell differentiation?
- <u>what</u> controls switch the DNAs' activities to meet the needs of the system at one time or another

(growth, repair, maintenance.., etc), or in the case of cancer, to challenge its wellbeing?

ENERGETIC MATRIX: PA-CO (PATTERN-CONTROL).

Let's examine the development of a system.

An organism starts at conception from a single cell containing one DNA. This *parent* cell divides in two and subsequent divisions brings the number of cells to about 2^n, n being the number of generations at maturity. An adult man has approximately $5 . 2^{12}$ cells. Here the proliferation stops and cell division occurs to replace cells in their normal turnover or to repair the accidental damage of tissues.

Consider the following situations:

1) The first DNA at conception carries the seed of evolutionary accomplishments up to the present human state, and to it is entrusted the full responsibility to produce the first generation of cells. It replicates **unaided, freely,** and the cell divides in response.

2) Two cells are born and the energetic pattern of the DNA daughters has already changed drastically for being *in company*. They *relate* to each other and the bond affects their decisions in the sense that now the DNAs' subordinate themselves to the energy of a *social relation*.

3) When division ends every DNA of each generation of cells relates to all other DNAs, all matter radiates energy. Assuming **one single** relation among two DNAs, the number of Class-1 relations responds to the formula:

r=number of relations

$$R= \frac{2^x (2^x - 1)}{2} \quad (A)$$

X=number of DNAs

(Class-1 bonds will generate the successive Class-2, Class-3, Class-4 ., etc to the final ones containing information from all DNAs. These ultimate bonds will integrate into one: the **will** of the system).

Even when the emanating energies shape into hierarchic structures, still formula (A) will represent a number far inferior to the total number of Class-1 DNAs relations in the system. I refer the reader to Chapter III for model's calculations.

Now let us analyze the energetic aspect of these Class-1 relations among DNAs.

Named E_T the total energy that one DNA has for its activities and E_e the minimum external energy DNA may expend on each relation, after X generation of cells, 2^x will be the number of DNAs and the total energy of relations E_T will be :

$$E_T = \frac{E_e \cdot 2^x (2^x - 1)}{2} \quad (1)$$

TABLE 3

(CLASS-1 DNAs' INTERRELATIONS)

No.generations; No.DNAs; No.relations; $\sum$ internal energies; $\sum$ relations' energies

1	2	1	$2 . E_i$	$1 . E_e$
2	4	6	$4 . E_i$	$6 . E_e$
3	8	28	$8 . E_i$	$28 . E_e$
4	16	120	$16 . E_i$	$120 . E_e$
:	:	:	:	:
:	:	:	:	:
x	2^x	$\dfrac{2^x(2^x-1)}{2}$	$2^x . E_i$	$\dfrac{2^x(2^x-1)}{2} E_e$
:	:	:	:	:
:	:	:	:	:
n	2^n	$\dfrac{2^n(2^n-1)}{2}$	$2^n . E_i$	$\dfrac{2^n(2^n-1) . E_e}{2}$ (1)

This amount increases extraordinarily with the number of generations for both factors 2^x and 2^x-1 grow exponentially with generations.

The energetic net or matrix of Class-1 interrelations at the last generation **n** of adulthood shall be named **PA-CO** for pattern-control. Each generation of DNAs will form its corresponding pattern-control. That is, at every stage of DNAs division a ***preliminary PA-CO*** will form in anticipation to the full development of the creature and a **PA-CO** will build upon **all** its Class-1 bonds.

Supposing that one DNA needs to function an internal energy $= E_i$ then $E_i = E_T - E_e$

The DNAs of generation X will have a total internal energy $= E_{ix} = E_i \cdot 2^x$ (2)

The rate between (1) and (2) will be:

$$E_e / E_i \cdot \frac{2^x (2^x - 1)}{2 \cdot 2^x} = E_e / E_i \cdot \frac{2^x - 1}{2}$$

This rate of PA-CO energy and internal energies of DNAs grows exponentially with the number of generations X as shows

$$\frac{2^x - 1}{2}$$

Eventually after a *critical number of divisions* the correspondent PA-CO will be greater than the internal energies of **all** DNAs, and being stronger will *control* (a better word would be *subordinate*) them. A simple quantitative reason. Therefore, the fate of DNAs -merely based in *quantitative* considerations- is to be controlled by PA-CO, the net of *interrelations' energies*.

With the progress of divisions this rate will increase and correspondingly the DNAs' subordination to their PA-CO also will increase. That means that in a creature development the emerging DNAs -at each succeeding generation of cells- are more disciplined than the previous ones, more socially entangled by reason only of energy-quantity. (Table 4 lists the PA-CO number of relations and energies here considered).

PA-CO AND DNA COMMUNICATION.

PA-CO energy, in addition, has an **intrinsic** controlling **quality,** and that is its *content of information*, which is superior to the content of information of DNAs individual energies. A second reason to effect DNAs subordination to the interrelations. This is a *qualitative* reason.

Communication among DNAs and PA-CO is a logical and inevitable event. Nor only it is possible but it is a consummated equilibrium. DNAs external energies coexist confined and satisfied among themselves in the DNAs energetic territorial limits. All them combined constitute **PA-CO** and this exerts control upon the DNAs of the system.

PA-CO and *individual DNAs energies* are on obvious communicating levels for **PA-CO** actually **is** *DNAs energies!*: internal and external (the external ones integrated in

PA-CO) and PA-CO receives, transfers and processes just the unaltered energy supplied by DNAs.

The conclusion is that: PA-CO has the capability to control DNAs imposing on them the social behavior carried within its integrated energetic pattern. And from the *successive PA-COs* evolved -along the creature development- and their control over DNAs derives the social enterprise of cell differentiation and cellular labor specialization.

The fact that a variety of body cells placed in a lab culture are able to selectively socialize is consistent with these views. First at all, matter has a social drive and sooner or later it will clearly manifest itself. Although cells of higher organisms when isolated are not under PA-CO control still they have been conditioned to a previous social behavior. This social tendency is strongly impressed on them to the point to appear in some instances out of their individual initiative. The spontaneous clustering of cells into fragments of the original tissues whence they proceed, as portions of liver or dermis, proves PA-CO's communication with DNAs, and that this communication got firmly imprinted in the genetic material to express itself even when out of the system.

TOTAL ENERGETIC STRUCTURE OF BIOSYSTEMS.

The PA-CO of each generation of cells is not static, it evolves Class-2, Class-3.., etc, bonds to the last ones with maximum control. And being such are evolvements of pure energy the total process takes place in a fraction of second. At same speed the evolving energetic bonds are forced into hierarchic patterns by the limits of reality. Physical dimensions constrict energies just as funnels channel and shape the fluids going through them.

Class-2 bonds and their matrix subordinate and communicate with Class-1 bonds and **PA-CO** in the same manner that these (Class-1 and **PA-CO**) relate to DNAs. That is, Class-2 and their matrix (pattern-control) have superior rank-control than **PA-CO** and its bonds. They are in *greater number* and their *content of information* is also superior to that of which they proceeded. Thus, they are in command of **PA-CO**. But nevertheless they should be able to communicate with PA-CO and its Class-1 bonds because the *information contained in Class-2 bonds is the combined information of two previous Class-1 bonds*. That is, both partake the same information or language.

The ascending energetic bonds and matrices relate to the preceding ones in equal fashion as those two first levels. Therefore, energy **control** is being secured by the automatic increase of informational content and amount of energy in the new-formed bonds and matrices. **Communication** also is insured *directly* among each **two consecutive levels** of bonds or energies because they co-share their information. The whole energetic castle of bonds and matrices up to the final ones shall be instantaneously created for their energies shall travel faster than the physical energy that they control. And this moves at light speed.

The previous reasoning establish the control of **PA-CO** over DNAs, but it can be seen that actually DNAs depend on the next energetic structure of bonds erected above PA-CO to which PA-CO is subordinated, and to the subsequent ones that subordinates the previous ones. Ultimately DNAs are subordinated, like the rest of the system, to the *integral control*: the WILL of the system. *Its decisions set the energetic state or pattern of the energetic castle.*

Most certainly the natural wisdom exhibited in the *visible and concrete world* is likewise operating under the *energetic realm* that regulates it. The energetic structure of biosystems is the perfect plan of the innumerable potential organizations conceivable notwithstanding that its creation is *instantaneous.* A few decades ago these energetic creations should have been rated as miracles. In today's computerized era of electronic speeds they are palpable realities. The speed and workings of the energetic castle of a biosystem, the unique jewel of eons of evolution, should not surprise us. Check yourself the energetic path of almost simultaneous *will to move* and resulting movement. The *will* shall convey its control to the energetic castle, which descend and translate this command level after level to the DNAs, which in turn preside the cellular activity of nerves and muscles that determine the move. And no energetic player misses the path.All is done in no time.

INCORRECT WIRED-IN INTERPRETATION.

The biosystems activities have been consistently interpreted by bio-science as *wired-in* processes along the physic-chemical action-reaction chains. A brief reflection makes obvious the foolishness of attempting to explain on these basis the integral functioning of creatures, specifically genetic activity. This methodology has already failed to explain the much simpler phenomena of the simultaneous symmetrical growth of crystals. How can it succeed in untangle a cellular organization as man whose proteins alone belong to about 10,000 types and in no place can be found the simplicity and regularity of crystal lattices?

The wired-in concept conflicts with the facts of which is of no minor importance the speed of bioreactions, and fails to explain the typical biological functions all of them based in *organic pattern*.

Memories illustrate these points. Creatures' learning are being printed and stored as soon as experimented, and can be recalled at any time of need or by *will*. It has been reported that cells' proteins increase their weight in the process of memorizing, and there is no *wired-in* mechanism that *connects one thought,* or feelings, *with DNAs*. This *wired-in* view excludes thoughts and feelings as subject matter of *physical* connections because they are not *concrete* reality. Memories of intelligent-emotional biosystems remain *unexplained*. During memorization the protein weight increases more prominently in brain cells but also occurs in somatic ones. No wired-in reaction explains the simultaneous printing of memories in 60 trillion cells that man has, nor the instant recall that implies the reversal of such protein formation to thought again...at wish.

Let's consider DNAs activities. The individualistic DNA, normal or cancerous, appears to resist or to be above all wired-in influence. In fact, no doctrine offers a model in the regulation of its behavior. *Wired-in* processes are time-dependent incapable to account for the permanent and orchestrated acting of DNAs having each the activity of one to one hundred million reactions per second.

With feedback regulation we encounter similar problems. This feedback loop has been discovered to work in a multitude of biological functions. Its operation though inescapably presupposes : 1) embodied *internal controls*, 2) *understandings*, and 3) *purposes*. These are not embraced in any way by the *wired-in* theories.

Electrical discharges of the brain and nerves are the main propellers of action. By which chained reactions to the very final causes are they generated? What stream of wired-in energy or combination of them contains the informational pattern of purpose and feeling? The answers are not there. *Wired-in* processes describe the *specifics* of *concrete* action-reaction. They have the value of a movie picture without answering for the integral, the general, the causative, or the intelligent planning.

The most indicting argument against the *wired-in* approach is that it fails to find the reasons for **control** and **subordination** that compels action, which includes the intercommunication and transformability among themselves of the prolific energies of biosystems. Informative content does not enter this conception, causes are left in the dark, and so typical biosystems' acts in the realm of the mysterious.

In contrast the theory of systems organizes this disjointed treatment into coherent framework by offering a **universal manner of action**. It places the *cause of action* on matter-energy, and deduces a *model of control-*

energies for systems' self-regulation. (That is, the regulation of all reality including biosystems.) This is another pending pivotal problem. Thus, the theory of systems, while gravitating the cause of action in matter-energy, retains *freedom of decision* to be the ultimate variable of the physical reality. The notion reconciles the initial action (cause of action due to elemental matter-energy) with the initiating of action by the system itself (cause of action in systems due to the integral control: the **will**.)

The energetic castle or matrix of the system functions instantaneously and the set of energy-controls determines *concrete* activities.

Decisions of the **wills** are unrelated to time and space. **Wills** do not travel. Each is an instant **yes** or **no** in situ, intransferable, a change of state that brings forth a change in the **wills-pattern** of the system. Not only the supreme **will** of the system but any **will**, however low in rank, in making a choice produces a new pattern with the innovation.

The pattern-change happens *at once*. The event is a quantum jump from one state to another. Nothing in between. No *wired-in* process involved. **Wills** do not develop. They are, or they are not. We see the universe moving and changing in relation of space-time. In relation to **wills** the energy the universe is closer to a film of incessant replacements, picture after picture, appearing and disappearing in infinitesimal pulsation, flickering at the sparkling of every elemental or complex decision. And they relate to the concrete via their infrastructure: the castle of control-energies whose **wills** also are deciders of states.

The concept of control-energies derives naturally from the phenomenon of association. Control-power is embodied in the informational content. Under this vision no distinctions of principle exists between the physical and the biological realities but one of degree that accounts for quality. Communication is feasible among all types of energy within the system thanks to its intertransformable processes. The theory of Systems, then, is the theoretical foundation of **CLINICAL BIOFEEDBACK** at **any biosystem level** down to the **genetic biofeedback** and **feedback at the elemental level of matter-energy**.

In the next CHAPTER we shall discuss that **PA-CO** is *instrumentally detectable* and the information it provides permits the actual control of the genetic machinery.

CHAPTER XII. – INTERPRETATION OF CANCER.

Systems do not welcome *imposed* forces and energies alien to the task to organize their realm. They are rejected as *hostilities*. The basic principles of the theory of natural systems does not admit another alternative because only the intelligence and freedom, ascribed to elemental matter-energy and systems, will work favorably for them. It is absolutely logical that the first encounter among *external controls* be one of rejection. Because the control cannot be recognized as self-control containing the information and the means to interpret it and decide for the self wellbeing. External compulsion is not only perceived as *hostile,* it is, in fact, *hostile*. The improbable occurrence that a benefit resulted by imposed control is a *chancy* one and in the chaotic immensity of the domain of *chance*

imposed controls invariably cause destruction of order, organization and structure.

This natural rejection compounded with the limitation of space might have accounted for the unimaginable violence of the universe in its first stages. Only superior energies created by associations, as described by this theory of systems, would have secured voluntary subordination and internal control, as it should be established in new systems. The original explosion might have provided the adequate distances for the subsistence of systems in that hostile environment.

Components are enticed and consolidated into stable unions by the *benefits* obtained walking in new paths that *while* integrating information, and because of said integration, create more intelligence and freedoms, and therefore more power! That is, <u>orders of higher capabilities</u> *shared by all the components*. Then such benefits trigger birth, life and the harmony of the new associations. Nevertheless no energy would integrate into another without organizing itself into powerful controls that would effect and preserve said integration.

Natural government has inherent *qualitative* and *quantitative* power over the governed by virtue of its superior information, and its greater amount of energy. After this government has been achieved, internal rejection of control totally disappears and the systems' components become receptive to the harmony, which they have contributed to create. Furthermore, such harmony gets impressed on them, they become conditioned to it, obedient to its designs even after separation of the system. The inanimate world expresses this by the resistance offered to an imposed change of state.

More sophisticated yet are the immune reactions of intelligent biosystems. They are their reactions to external control and damage caused by it. Biosystems have the *information* for proper functioning and preservation, and no external advisor, orders and organizations can substitute their *intelligence* in solving their problems. No external *energies or controls* can improve the government of the energetic castle erected harmoniously from the minutest elemental energy-quantum up to the end product, the **integral will,** because this is based on the system's intelligence and its informed decisions.(I will write **WILL** when referring to this **integral will**).

If cancer were indeed an exclusive affair of the DNA there would be no sensible excuse for lack of self-correction or failure to trigger its mechanisms of self-repair. These mechanisms have been verified to exist by electronic microscopy. And the worse part, *cancer would be incurable,* for there is no molecule, natural or synthetic, or combination of them, able to supply the colossal amount of information that DNA uses in its own restoration. A *wonder drug* of this caliber is and will be forever beyond science's capabilities.

The development of human DNA took evolution ages of work in the best-equipped laboratory, Nature itself! Besides the synthesis of *free and intelligent* controls that go along with it, human DNA needs the guidance of PA-CO energy, which also cannot exist apart from the energetic castle of the creature. The endeavor to synthesize such *wonder drug* embraces an immense number of theoretical impossibilities and *absolutely needed knowledge out of reach* -starting with the Heisenberg principle of uncertainty for elemental particles- but, in addition, infinite impossibilities of *action* for man cannot create *free decisions* upon which these *actions* are propelled. Natural freedom to decide is granted by the grace of God, the same source from which matter and energy arrived to the Creation. To those opposing this notion, one may ask: Is it not more amazing the arrival of matter-energy than the arrival of their baggage of freedom and intelligence?

Fortunately, cancer is not a DNA's problem in spite to the fact that the item deemed to be cancerous or not cancerous is DNA. Cancer is a body dysfunction that irremediably causes the body's death while DNA will continue living in one way or another. An *order* -as the body of the cancer patient- that runs to its destruction is the one that has the problem and its possible solution because it knows its organization and has the resources to maintain and restore it again when it has not been irreversible damaged.

Notice that the theory of systems approaches the functioning of systems *at the energetic level,* which constitutes the program that matter will follow. A healthy body is supported by an harmonious castle of energies where minor energy disharmonies, as those produced by an unruled DNA, have a short life in the dimensions of light-speed energy. A body with a healthy energetic pattern should promote DNAs' energetic harmony and therefore DNAs' and cells' healthy functioning.

THE CURE OF CANCER.

Genetic errors do arise inevitably in the development of a creature and during the several decades of its life-span. The number of replications of DNA in this period is a *staggering figure* and its normal activity is of the order of one million to one hundred million reactions *each second.* It is rather inconceivable that a system of such vertiginous and intricate action be free of error moreover when every element is a *free* decider. Genetic mistakes do occur frequently and are corrected by the alert responses of the DNAs or the powerful responses of the castle of energy that presides DNAs' actions. One may assume too the altruism and elimination of the useless DNAs for the wellbeing of the

279

body, as social insects accept self-sacrifice as part of their social duties. We know that routinarily the body eliminates unnecessary materials. It is the conflicting meaning in DNAs' programming, the extent of the sacrifice demanded, or the persistence of damaging stimuli, that may pose sufficient threat for *one DNA* to resort to uncontrolled cancerous behavior. The reason being that DNA is essentially a code of life and deprived of proper social guidance it would follow its code of unstopping reproduction.

It is obvious that the cancer problem is not a *local one* considering that the *inductive forces of surrounding healthy DNAs* cannot reverse the cancerous spring of that *single DNA.* The problem is more *general.* DNA's immunity in that cancerous DNA is deficient because genetic defenses are already deficient at the PA-CO level that should have induced DNA to a program of recovery.

That any DNA can be the target of cancer without specific reason to account for, and the unpredictability of cancer's location, point to the same conclusion: that PA-CO is the *cancerous* blue print and the one in need to be restored to a pattern of genetic harmony. When this is accomplished PA-CO will be in the position to promote DNAs' social behavior and to oblige cancerous DNAs to undergo the proper adjustments to comply with it. Those DNAs beyond repair will follow the usual course of elimination by apt immune defenses.

The loss of PA-CO healthy social and immune programs leaves erroneous DNAs in conflict with other healthy DNAs, with no map to join organized tissues, and at the mercy of its own resources, its nucleotides' codes, which dictate the reproduction of individualistic cells into unorganized tumors. Thus, cancer is not due to a *cancerous DNA* but to a *cancerous PA-CO*.

In short: the restoration of a cancerous PA-CO to a genetically healthy pattern is the cure of cancer. The **Will** has the power and the information to do this restoration if it receives the proper genetic feedback information.

Summarizing:

1) The self-repair of the DNA is *the only possible way* to turn cancerous DNA into healthy DNA and should be the aim of research instead of a search for the unreachable *wonder drug* or *external cure*. Genetic immunity is a natural process, it is specifically DNA's work! Cancerous DNA contains the adequate information to reverse to its healthy state. Neither lab techniques nor molecules can do the job that belongs to the DNA by its own constitution.

2) PA-CO pattern promotes genetic harmony and when this is disrupted it has the power to induce and re-establish social order. Per force cancerous DNAs will mobilize their immune resources and healing power. Those DNAs beyond repair, threatening the wellbeing of

the body, will be eliminated with the *precision* of the body's inductive energies that no surgery can match nor chemotherapies or radiotherapies have.

Before proceeding let's see whether there is empirical medical support to embark on this course of research.

CLINICAL BIOFEEDBACK.

Some organs and mechanisms of the body seem to work automatically without conscious effort. Kidneys, heart, cells, circulation of blood and nutrients, thermoregulation, and immune reactions are not attended by the mind. Others respond to direct commands of the **Will** as they are movements, speech, and mental work.

Observation of these differences shaped a unanimous consensus, prevalent until 50 years ago, that the body's functions fall into two distinct categories, voluntary and involuntary, whether or not they were under the **Will**'s control.

The doctrine that elements or functions cannot be controlled by **Will** has been progressively discarded with the advances of instrumentation. One by one the involuntary labels have been erased, as therapies using voluntary control had been developed. The illusion of lack of control was due to the lack of feedback information. When the connection **Will** to **results** is made available, the sense of control is regained. Control always was there, although, not the way to detect this control. These therapies are common today in most hospitals under the name of CLINICAL BIOFEEDBACK, which entitles the control of *physiological functions* at **Will** when simultaneous feedback information is given to the patient by instrumentation.

FOUNDATION OF CLINICAL BIOFEEDBACK.

The theory of systems gives a *theoretical foundation* of these successful medical practices. It postulates, deduces –and is supported by abundant medical evidence– that **the Will of a system**, the human body in this case, has the control, decides for the system, and subordinates the **wills** of each of its elements. (Notice that I refer to these as **wills** to distinguish them from the **Will** of system).

A person that chooses to jump from the Washington Bridge, will end with all his DNAs in the river. The control of his **Will** over the whole body is obvious in this case. But, what about the *specific* subordination of the **wills** of each element of the body? Yes, the **integral Will** is also vested with such power embodied in the total harmony of the energetic castle. The energetic castle subordinates each DNA, and ultimately the DNAs preside the cellular activity of each and every body's function. The control is *specific* and *total* for it is built on a *continual* creation of *specific* energy-controls in ascending degree of power from the DNAs energies to the highest level of energy, the **Will**. No energies other than the ones generated by the process of bonding are needed or are possible. Each *state* of the energetic castle is unique and enacted by the ultimate variable, the free decision of the **integral Will,** and this *state* determines total and specific actions.

The **Will** has the energetic connections to subordinate each component, although not in the wired-in fashion. Moreover, not only one act of the **Will** translates into an energetic pattern of the whole castle instantaneously, but also the **will** of a mere element is never an isolated event. It sets also *a state* on the creature's energies and, regardless of the infinitesimal change it may represent, it also sets *a state* in the entire universe. According to this point of view the *specificity* of the pattern is what promote the *specific* action of each element.

Let's go to the medical proofs of **unicellular** control by the **will**.

CLINICAL BIOFEEDBACK AT THE CELLULAR LEVEL.

Dr. B. Brown in her book NEW MIND, NEW BODY[2] devotes some 40 pages (Chapter V) to the *voluntary control* of a single cell.

The basic research conducted by Dr. J. V. Basmajian is detailed on several papers[3] where he describes and proves the control of one neuromotor cell not only by conscious **Will** but also by the subconscious **will**.

With a cathode ray oscilloscope and a small electrode sensor of 25 micromillimeters diameter he tapped electrical voltages fired by muscle cells and translated them into visual versions either by a recording-pen on a moving graph-paper, with coordinates microvolts versus milliseconds, or into images on an oscilloscopic screen. The signals reflect, with its ups and downs, the electrical discharges during muscle activity and rest.

Each motor unit is composed of a *group of muscular cells* and *one single nerve-cell* that activates them. The instantaneous information obtained from these units allows the subject to *voluntarily* control his muscle activity and therefore the *single nerve-cell that enervates it*! A variety of subjects including children under six years of age and mental patients have been proven capable to be trained in *single nerve-cell* control, in about twenty minutes. What is really outstanding is that the training is enhanced with better understanding of the experiments. The control extends to situations where the action of the muscle unit is carried out while the consciousness is busy doing other tasks like having a TV interview or playing an instrument. In this situation the cell is then influenced only by the

subconscious Will that apparently has a prominent role in the control of the body.

<u>CELLULAR CONTROL. - SIGNIFICANCE.</u>

The salient features of the research are:

1) Control of the production and inhibition of the motor-unit. It is interesting to note that the activity-signals of a muscle can be controlled but the **shape** of such signals that is characteristic of each particular unit **cannot.**

2) Control of *one single nerve-cell* upon command of the **Will.**

3) Identification by the **conscious or subconscious Will** of <u>one</u> out of ten billion nerve-cells in the brain hemisphere where the cell is located.

4) Control over the simultaneous functions needed to *activate* the nerve-cell and to *inhibit* many others.

5) Acquisition of a *learned conditioning* that makes feedback control progressively easier.

Conscious understanding of the technique highly improves and shortens the time of training.

6) Learned control also influences the speed of control-learning to **unrelated** cells. (When one side of the body is trained, the training of the other side becomes easier).

The whole phenomenon is caused by the *internal* controls of the body, the *specific* patterns set by the energetic castle. No other explanation is possible. Of another totally different character are the physic-chemical reactions that generate the electrical discharges. These are typical *external* actions among hierarchic factions *not sharing information*, and a consequence of the body being a system of systems hierarchically structured.

The transcendental conclusions to be drawn from Dr. Basmajianm's research are that the **conscious or subconscious Will** exerts control over *one single cell*, *identifies* it among billions of them, and is all done in a *fraction of a second*.

Compare the efficiency of this control with the difficulties an expert finds seeking one particular electrical wire among billions, if that is needed for a repair (surely the repair will never be done). You will see the superiority of internal-control over the external control man shall exert in his dealings with the world. In addition, if you consider that such internal control is *intranferable*, you will have an idea of the *privileged powers* that each system has in controlling its functioning.

Until now the experiments of single-cell control demonstrated some crucial matters of monumental importance: 1) The connection between **Will** (*abstract energy*) and **cell** (*concrete matter-energy*), 2) The supreme rank-control of the **Will** (in the body's hierarchic structuration) that embraces *cellular specificity* (selectivity and timing) that implies **genetic specificity** as DNA presides cellular activity, and 3) The extreme resistance to change the shape-graph of the motor unit - in all practicality its autograph- which proves a *natural* resistance to malfunction.

Now, let's go to the cause of events.

CAUSE OF CELLULAR CONTROL.

Conscious Will resides at the top of the energetic castle, so to speak. **Subconscious Will** should occupy some place on it also. The brain activity that stimulates the single *nerve-cell* while inhibiting others is a *simultaneous* event, one grounded in the activities of the brain's DNAs, which in turn respond to the patterned guidance of PA-CO, at once. At the other end of the process there are the *muscle's DNAs* activating the responses of the muscle cells unit. Such responses are characteristic signatures of each motor cell despite being the nerve's stimulus **one** and the **same** for *various groups of cells*, for it is *one single neuron* that serves several families of muscles-cells. These muscle DNAs are also guided by PA-CO, and alot of intermediate reactions along the route brain-muscle are activated too by their corresponding DNAs. Therefore, these experiments lead inescapably to conclude that the cause of action is born in the **Will,** propagates throughout the energetic castle to the PA-CO level that takes care of DNAs' activity from head to toe and in between every body's segment.

Wired-in theories do not explain the *simultaneousness* of the functions involved, the learning and conditioning, the distant induction by the *learned* cells, or the improvement of training by the *conscious understanding* it. In fact, the very connection of the **Will** (abstraction) **-cell** (matter) cannot be answered by wired-in reactions that only occur among concrete realities. The answers belong to the *energetic dimension* whose macro-concrete effects are those <u>physiological</u> results, those <u>wired-in</u> electrical discharges between hierarchically separated physical realities.

Dr. Brown mentioned in her book (New Mind, New Body) the <u>*natural asynchrony* of muscle cells reactions</u>, a precision coordinated mechanism of firings absolutely needed to avoid muscular rigidity. Asynchrony cannot be controlled at **Will** *except for a very few seconds!* Although these few seconds prove the integral control of the **Will,** yet this resistance to control is equivalent to an **immune reaction at the genetic level**. It practically resists **Will-control** of time-functioning of an order **below microseconds** when those imposing timings are damaging the health of the system.

LIMITS OF THE WILL.- ENERGETIC EQUILIBRIUMS.

The picture of the energetic castle is becoming clearer with these empirical findings. On the one side, they tell us that the **Will** has supreme power over the **specific** and the **whole**. On the other, they unveil the facts that the body offers resistance to the **Will** when it acts against the health of the system, like tampering with the muscular asynchrony or with the shapes of the oscillographic lines obtained by Dr.Basmajian. The body that heals wounds that have been *voluntarily* inflicted upon it conveys the same message. The healing is a genetic immune reaction counteracting the effects of a destructive conscious **Will**.

Notice that the energetic castle appears to act as a republic limiting the absoluteness of power of the *integral* **Will** with the wills-equilibrium of the rest of the energies that have established the harmony of the system.

The theory of systems is universal, it applies to elemental matter-energy as well as to all systems. It postulates that concrete reality operates *democratically* not only inside of the system but across the entire universe for the universe qualifies too as a system, the all encompassing system. Free acting across the spectrum of the Creation drives towards universal wills-equilibrium and harmony! There is no doubt in my mind that American Republic owes its stability for being in accord with the general laws of Nature.

If the success of Clinical Biofeedback is actually related to its understanding, the theory of systems would greatly improve and expand the frontiers of feedback therapies in muscular and nerve rehabilitation and similar treatments because *it provides an explanation* of the foundation and mechanisms of Clinical Biofeedback.

HABITUAL CONTROL OF DNAS.

Unaware of it, man is continuously controlling and manipulating his DNAs because DNAs are obeying, getting damaged or being repaired in their fantastic interweaving with PA-CO. PA-CO responds to the overpowering energy castle, which is under the sovereign power of the **Will.**

PA-CO is a more powerful reality than the DNAs. We have already persistently stressed this point. It is the general law of evolution. The result of association overrules the cause, the associates. That causes creation and new orders.

The simple act to blink an eye goes beyond the DNAs actions to generate cellular nerve and muscular eye blinking. It means that PA-CO has set the DNAs into those particular actions. To lift a hand is done with the cooperative effort of many DNAs that activate muscular and nerve cells to that end, but behind this effort is the actual inducing push of PA-CO energy. Nerve, muscle stimulation and every body's game resting among the 60 trillion DNAs has its start in PA-CO, but in essence and in all cases the **Will**, conscious or unconscious, controls PA-CO. To conjure cancer, AIDS and genetic disorders is not the exclusive doing of DNAs. The **Will** pre-ordains the system's physiological doings via the progressive demotion of its powers along the energetic castle, PA-CO, DNAs and cells.

The marvelous structure and operation of systems is intended primarily to preserve the system's well being. Disasters may happen where errors are possible, and when they do, still the tremendous army of DNAs is designed to mobilize a plan of correction of abnormalities under the guidance of PA-CO via the energetic castle and under the **Will**. The **Will** holds the reins of GENETIC ACTIVITY, at each fraction of a second! One tiny rebellious DNA has no chance of escaping the control of the body and the inductive forces of 60 trillion healthy DNAs. It is the **Will** that is responsible for the well functioning of DNAs and also for their wrong functioning. Our own **will** is a tool of awesome power to be mightily feared. When wrongly used it can disrupt the whole genetic machinery, and this is far more dangerous, than not to discern food from poison.

To understand that the **Will** controls or induces DNAs is to hit upon one of the main causes of ailments: the patient himself. To discover the proper use of **Will-control** over DNAs is to discover the most general, efficient and safest cure of disease, GENETIC HEALING. How can this goal be achieved? There is only one path: GENETIC BIOFEEDBACK.

GENETIC BIOFEEDBACK.

In order for the patient *to relate* the speedy changes of the DNAs (at 10^{-6} to 10^{-8} of a second) to the changes of the **Will,** the feedback information should be *instantaneous* and *precise.* That makes the project altogether impossible.

No instrumentation seems feasible to check individual activities of the DNAs in vivo. Medical devices can hardly cope with diagnosis of clearly declared tumors or genetic problems, and samples shall be extracted from the body. This process requires time and, as said, genetic information shall be instantaneous. The extreme complexity of genetic reactions, the microdimensions of molecules, the extraordinary number of DNAs, the arbitrary nature of cancer weigh all the more against any *direct* instrumental detection that could be adopted for Clinical Biofeedback of DNAs behavior.

The enterprise to develop feedback instrumentation at the genetic level must take another route: Detection of PA-CO states, identification of PA-CO patterns -that induce genetic health or genetic abnormalities- and manipulation and restoration of the unhealthy PA-CO pattern to normality, that is, to healthy PA-CO pattern that reflects the body's harmony above and below it. Let's examine the theoretical and empirical grounds for this research.

CHARACTER OF PA-CO PATTERN.

From the theory of systems it follows:

1) Only PA-CO contains the *total guidance* of DNAs and the ability *to communicate* it to the *DNAs*.

2) The changes of PA-CO are *instantaneous* across the whole PA-CO pattern. Actually any change across the whole energetic castle defining a *new state* is completed in no time

3) Changes are *total*. There are no changes on parts, or sections of the PA-CO pattern . There are *states* of equilibrium. An alteration of **one** DNA should be reflected in the PA-CO pattern or in any partial expression of it.

4) The **Will** decides and sets the *total state* of the energetic castle and this is reflected on the PA-CO pattern.

MATERIALIZATION AND DEMATERIALIZATION.

Let us examine internal energies in relation to their instrumental detection. To do that we shall succinctly analyze the process of abstraction of *concrete* energies to *undetectable* ones within the system.

To *see* an object, for instance a flower, is to *print it* on the retina as a photographic machine would do. The *sensorial print* is a **concrete molecular** reality. Automatically without conscious effort this print is converted, by whatever workings or associations of energies may occur, into a *image*, some kind of representation of the lines, shape, volume, etc., of *that* particular flower and no other one. The *image's energy* travels; it is stored some place *out of the retina*, very likely in all DNAs, from where it may be recalled *at will*. (An increase of weight had been observed in the proteins of the brain during the process of learning or memorizing). The image is a superior structure to the sensorial print, due to the processing that the print undergoes to create it. Body energies, as every other energy do not stop. Energy continues traveling and associating continuously into new energies, new orders. Subsequently, and perhaps after seeing several other flowers, the mind forms the *idea* of a flower. The **idea** is a more complex pattern of energy than the **image** is. Obviously so because it embraces not *one* flower, but *all* flowers, even those *not yet seen!* That implies far more information and therefore superior energy. The new entity **-idea-** has the power to *recognize* any flower whatsoever to be a flower, without relation to color, shape or volume. It is an **abstraction** devoid of any *concrete* features, not even representation of them.

Thus, the above sequence shows that the *process of abstraction* requires the evolvement and creation of superior energy. Sensorial print, image, idea, are each one energetically more complex, more informed, and more intelligent than the preceding ones and, for this very reason, superior to them. But, at the same time, they are less and *less instrumentally detectable* for they are no longer *concrete* items to be detected. The flower is a *concrete* creature, the sensorial print a *molecular* reality, the image a *mental* representation that we may be able to reproduce in a drawing or simply to remember by extracting it from the DNAs' energies. But the **idea** has lost *all physical features*. It has no form no color, no weight to describe, nothing that limits its capability. It comprehends all possible flowers present, past or future ones, which adds to the mystery of abstraction. Most flowers are not part of the information that created the idea. It is enough to say that when internal energies become more complex ones they also become more abstract, *more independent of physical agents* and therefore *more undetectable by instrumentation.*

As illustrated above on *ideas* evolving from *vision*, biosystems have mechanisms to transform concrete energies into abstract ones and viceversa. *Undetectable* energies will de-escalate, by dislodging their bonds and content of information, to become simpler energies that may communicate with concrete reality either concrete energy or concrete matter. This process of *dematerialization or abstraction* takes place in the energetic castle at the formation of Class-1 bonds, Class-2 bonds, Class-3 bonds up to the **Will**. The opposite, *materialization*, shall happen for the **Will** to become and communicate with *detectable* energy. We don't know what Class of bonds are instrumentally detectable but we can fairly assume that PA-CO, the Class-1 bonds of the DNAs' energies, **IS**, for it communicates with all and each DNA to guide their social activity. If PA-CO affects DNA, which is a molecule, a **concrete** reality, observable, measurable, for the same reasons it shall affect other **concrete** realities.

Theoretically it is possible to detect the *external energies* of the DNAs and according to deductions 1 to 4 on page 295 said detection shall allow us to tap PA-CO (energy-pattern) energy or whatever expression of it that may tell *its state, which is the total net of DNAs' external energies.*

Because of these same premise, the calibration of a suitable instrumentation that would detect any aspect of

PA-CO, and therefore of the healthy or unhealthy state of the castle of energies, should not offer difficulties. It would simply require a preliminary work of collecting data from healthy people and from patients with specific ailments and/or degree of them. And, as in any biofeedback technique, the subject after adequate training should be able to trigger PA-CO healthy patterns **at Will**. That is, he should be able to re-program DNAs from cancerous behavior to healthy one, or from any other disease to normality according to how the instrumentation has been calibrated.

Should the tapping of PA-CO energy by instrumentation be achieved, medicine may undergo two new developments: 1) to cure most diseases at the *genetic* level by GENETIC BIOFEEDBACK (all diseases have a genetic origin or component) rather than at the *physiological* level by external remedies or physical amputation, and 2) to cure the *typically genetic diseases,* as cancer, which until now could not be cured because no methodology was available to re-program or induce the repair the DNAs at **WILL**.

CHAPTER XIII. - ORGANIZING THE EXTERNAL.

We have analyzed how **will**, an *undetectable* energy, might control the system by *internal* energies and internal processes. The **will** undergoes a degradation of energy via the successive splitting of bonds, descending from Class to Class to every level of energy and finally reaching the DNA, a concrete reality.

One shall assume that the energies of a system will not communicate among themselves without a transformation that provides for an equivalent informational content. Obviously, *undetectable* energies cannot communicate directly with *concrete* reality. There is no point of contact or common language.

Experience also shows that systems induce *external* order on less organized systems and that such order is directly related to the *internal* order of the system. Atoms impose order in energy flowing throughout their orbitals by absorbing and emitting specific quantities of it. The energies absorbed or emitted are *external* orders that accurately reflect the *internal* atomic structure in the spectrographic lines of absorption or emission. Any atom can be identified by its spectrographic lines despite being located in a star a thousand light-years away. A seed crystal in a solution of its ions forces them to move in its direction. Very uncomplicated, but *that* is an *order*. The ions are under the seed's control. Molecules or molecular systems create intricate *external* orders in proportion to their informational content (quantitative as well as qualitative), which is to say, to their intelligence. This external power escalates in biosystems.

With a little mental effort we can separate various levels of energies within a single biosystem and visualize that each one may have its own particular organizational power over *external* elements and systems, provided that said power be transformed into concrete energy compatible with the external physical reality.

The *exterior* can be organized by the top level of energy, the **integral-Will-energy**. This highest, most complex energy carries out operations in the *external* world by *external* action, and the orders it produces reflect the highest intelligence of the biosystem. That action is clearly preceded by a previous transformation of the *undetectable will* to the *concrete energies* of

DNAs. DNAs ultimately act upon cells and these cells upon *concrete* external reality. Thus, human beings project innumerable orders of every kind, practical, social, artistic, scientific, moral, etc.., by *external* control. My **Will**, for instance, has allowed me to write this booklet by using information and the means to organize it at the level of physical reality.

Leaving aside the **Will**, human judgment, and the rest of conscious acts, other energies of the biosystem most certainly control the environment in the practice of self-supporting, forcing *orders* on external elements. But no piece of art, book or code of ethics will come from these subordinated **wills** or energies. Their *induced orders* are a reflection of their energies and controls, which depend on information and intelligence. No group of cells, however gifted can compose a symphony, a piece of legislation or a moral precept. A subordinated **will** lacks the energy, information and intelligence required by these tasks. The *orders* they project outside of the system will not be a Shakespearean play, rather a play reflecting their endeavors and *states* induced by the particular **control-will** of that energy.

The *external* orders that PA-CO energy may originate, we will call **external genetic orders**, are the ones that we must attempt to tap if we intend to see the relation between the **conscious Will** and its effect on the programming of DNAs. Such information will allow the development of **Genetic Biofeedback.** The reasons to tap PA-CO and no other level of energy are given below.

EXTERNAL GENETIC ORDERS.

The *external orders* that we intend to use for Genetic Clinical Biofeedback are caused by altogether different types of energies than the ones recorded by Dr.Basmajian in his one-cell control experiments. His graphs represent *wired-in* processes, local electrical discharges between the nerve and the muscular cells, which are *concrete* energies that do not share their contents of information. They are particular physiological effects resulting from the cells' activity after being activated by *selected* DNAs' programs applied to one or another cell. PA-CO had directed DNAs to act differently in muscle cells than in nerve cells. The *physiological* results and the electrical discharges, do not contain the complete make up of the DNA, and much less the one of the PA-CO pattern of energies that assigns specific jobs to each DNA. Their energies are inferior to PA-CO and even to DNAs energy levels.

In **Genetic Biofeedback** we are looking for direct information from PA-CO, this **patterned social order, this total energy-matrix** that induces and guides – **at once**– the entire cellular complex. Electrical discharges of muscle units do not have such information.

Muscles and cells are already hierarchic *subsystems* each incapable of containing the vast PA-CO information that represents the *whole genetic control*. Cells *know* how to behave in the context of other cells not by their content of information, or the content of information of their DNAs, that is the same in all cells, but because they communicate with the clearinghouse PA-CO, the satellite that decides and transmits the *selected* program that their DNAs shall run. Equally unsuitable to our purpose are the patterns of brain activity given by the BEAM (Brain Electrical Activity Mapping) machines. This approach is again the detection of *wired-in* reactions among independent cells. The 20 electrodes applied around the areas of the head check electrical signals fired by brain neurons. The map of firing-rates does not say anything about the total PA-CO control-map over the cells.

EEGs (Electroencephalogram) are in the same category. They are recordings of subsystems' electromagnetic activities. And, in general, the entire field of present medical instrumentation has been conceived and developed on the bases of *wired-in* processes. These types of phenomena serve well Clinical Biofeedback *at the muscular and nerve levels* but cannot be used for **Clinical Genetic Biofeedback** that seeks the effect of **Will-decisions** upon the DNAs. The strings of the *genetic* drama belong to PA-CO and in the tapping of PA-

CO pattern of energy rests the foundation of **Genetic Biofeedback.** The *external genetic orders* that tell its *state* and can be used as feedback information are those directly **induced** by PA-CO.

Undetectable energies are not energetic orders of the sort of sound or other manifestations of the spectrum of electromagnetic waves, which includes radio, TV, infrared, visible, UV, X-Rays, gamma waves, etc.., up to cosmic rays. The reason has been repetitively and categorically presented: *these energies have no concrete dimensions*, and they cannot interact with *concrete* reality such as electromagnetic waves. They should be transformed via processes within the bioenergetic castle into PA-CO energies, and once they are embodied in PA-CO, they can order, or induce order on physical matter-energy. Because PA-CO interacts with DNAs that are *concrete*, molecular realities; they also will interact with other *concrete* physical realities. No such thing can be said of the levels of energy above that of PA-CO, for they are no longer simple bonds of DNAs energies but rather more complex ones, with increased quality and amount of energy that in their evolvement have become instrumentally *undetectable*.

PA-CO's induced orders over external reality reflect its own pattern, and its *state-changes* under the mandate of the **Will.** But there is another fundamental reason why PA-CO patterns are the proper information in genetic feedback, and that is, the *vertiginous speeds* of the castle of energies and DNAs' reactions. Genetic feedback information shall be almost simultaneous in order to relate *one* decision of the **Will** with the *genetic change* it produces, otherwise, no one could relate *that* decision to *that* change. Physiological **Will** decisions to serve as biofeedback information upon which to correct the action of the **Will**. We are interested in controlling the DNAs' programs and DNAs repair mechanisms before they trigger the subsequent cellular functions.

The problem of detection of PA-CO is greatly simplified by the fact that Genetic Clinical Biofeedback is centered in the **changes of pattern** (not in elucidating its structure) under the influence of **Will**.

DETECTION OF GENETIC EXTERNAL ORDERS.

The research here proposed is **to single out genetic external orders induced by PA-CO and select a variable in them that respond to PA-CO changes of state.** Other external orders or manifestations interfering with these PA-CO orders shall be eliminated or minimized.

PA-CO and DNAs energies affect every energy that cross our planet for this is precisely what biological energies are habitually doing, choosing and controlling their surroundings in the manufacturing and maintenance of their bio-organizations. Their control extends to electromagnetic energies, elemental particles and systems, on the basis of their *superior rank* of control and intelligence.

Space is permeated by an immense variety of energies: sound, gravity, and in general electromagnetic radiation covering wave ranges of 0.0001 Å (Angstrom =one hundred millionth of a cm.) to 100 Km. and given the limitations of instrumental detection probably beyond these limits. This thesis increases this range of energies with the countless *energy-controls* it postulates. *Control-energies* and their induced orders have not been introduced to science, but recognition of them promises to be in sight soon considering the speedy accumulation of data by computers.

STIMULATION OF BIOSYSTEMS' EXTERNAL ORDERS.

The energy that matter radiates, as to the type of projected energy and the patterns that external elements may adopt, varies with the sort of stimulation it receives. A piece of metal for instance, will radiate different light colors when heated at different temperatures, or will merely emit heat, sound or electricity under other conditions. Metals have a more stable structure than biosystems and the energetic output and induced orders mainly vary in relation to the stimulus, if the metal does not get contaminated or its shape altered. When it does, then the external pattern would differ from the previous one assuming these alterations. Afterwards the new pattern would be stable again. Induction of external orders or emission of energies is thus marked by *order* responding to both the *inductors and the stimulus' orders*. Radiation and induced external order produced by inanimate matter -whether or not stimulated- are fruitful fields for the exploration of the structure of matter, atomic or molecular, and in general of systems and their functions.

Equally, energetic stimulation of biosystems may improve the detection of their external orders on concrete reality. That is, external orders that are *not* instrumentally detectable at first attempt may be made detectable by providing certain matter-energy to the biosystem that enable it to enhance such induced orders. The difficulty of singling out the external orders produced by PA-CO, which should be very characteristic, can be solved in any event. **Research in this field is most urgent given the palpable limitations of present medical treatments in dealing with *genetic healing*.**

POTENTIAL TECHNIQUES FOR GENETIC EXPLORATION.

Two considerations are to be taken in the stimulation of biosystems to induce external orders suitable for instrumental detection: 1) The stimulant energy shall not be injurious to the biosystem. 2) It shall accentuate specifically the PA-CO inducted order while avoiding stimulation of other energies whose induction may conflict or obscure the PA-CO induced order.

One technique that produces a rich spectrum of energetic bio-information is the application of high voltage, high frequency electromagnetic radiation to biosystems. (Frequencies over 10^4 Hz., voltages about 5,000 to 40,000 volts of alternating current). Frequencies below 10^4 Hz. are detrimental to bio-organisms. This and higher frequencies are safer because they travel on the outer surface of conductors and because they exceed the upper frequency limits of nerve and muscle tissues. The energetic manifestations are visible in the form of coronas around the object.

Electrotherapies have been used for more than two centuries and though the luminosity produced by high frequency currents had been observed long before, not until 1939 was it photographed for the first time in Russia by Semyon D. Kirlian and his wife Valentina. They earnestly took this project at heart and devoted most of their life to film these suggestive images whose nature remains until now a matter of inconclusive interpretation.

Kirlian photography does not use any lighting other than the one coming from the object under observation stimulated by high frequency, high voltage electromagnetic radiation, which has been proven to be safe when applied to biosystems.

From the Kirlian photographs it was soon realized: 1) that the luminescent haloes and coronas appearing in the process show *shapes and patterns* clearly distinct from magnetic and electric ones, 2) that coronas of living systems have structural details which those of non-living objects lack, and 3) that intensively vivid coronas of living organizations such as a freshly plucked leaf gradually fades when life withers, and totally disappears in time. These observations point to the conclusion that the Kirlian patterns are related to the typical biological function that we name life. Apparently the aura of a human finger is altogether different from that obtained from the finger of a surgical glove filled with water at body's temperature, or the finger of a dead person. The differences are not only in shape and structure but also in dynamism. This last aspect may have inspired author Kendall Johnson to title a book about these induced orders: THE LIVING AURA (1975).

Pioneers of Kirlian techniques in USA are Dr. Thelma Moss (Neuropsychiatry Institute of the University of California, Los Angeles), Psychiatrist Montague Ullman (Maimonides Medical Center, New York), William A. Tiller (Stanford University, Stanford. California. Department of Materials, Science & Engineering), Dr. Stanley Krippner (Dream Laboratory, Maimonides Medical Center, New York).

Throughout the years curiosity has spread; investigators and techniques multiplied yielding exciting printings with a prolific variety of images, color and responses. While the mystically inclined sees in the Kirlian corona the flaring of the *astral* body predicated by eastern beliefs, the *wired-in* minded scientist identifies the effect with *ionic collisions* due to electrons emitted by the biosystem, and nothing else.

The implication that *non-physical* energies (the astral bodies) are *directly* photographed is plainly absurd. How can *undetectable* energies without any concrete feature *collide* with the photographic film when such ghosts are supposed to go through thick walls without the least inconvenience? Joking aside, only *external* energies of the DNA, a *concrete* molecule, can interact with *concrete* matter-energy. There is no avenue for the sequence of materialization to dematerialization and viceversa other than that performed by the castle of energies via association and disassociation of its bonds-energy. Their association gives origin to an increase of the quantity and quality of the bond-energy, and the opposite happens in their disassociation.

Nevertheless, regardless of the vagueness of the *astral* concept and absurd claim that non-physical energies are directly detected on film, this *holistic view* that reads in bioluminescence a reflection of *inner states* is much closer to reality than the *wired-in* one. The wired-in approach, in trying to dissect and precisely describe reality, ironically misses *the pattern of the whole* and by this, it does not comprehend nor explain the complete and typical functions of biosystems. It stands on defective and incomplete ground: the components and their *external* interrelations, which are in fact a consequence of the total castle of energies totally omitted by said approach.

Dr. S. Prat and J. Schemmer reported that in the corona obtained from plant leaves can be found infrared, visible and UV radiations. Auras still appear when filters impermeable to these radiations were placed between the leaves and the film. (Journal of Biological Photographic Assoc. June 1930 pg. 145-148). Dr. Moss, attempting to elucidate the *nature* of Kirlian coronas, screened all radiations of wavelength from UV through infrared and she still obtained a picture of a leaf though a very much dimmer one.

Obviously if **all** radiations were screened there would be no picture at all for lack of matter-energy to be ordered by biological induction. Kirlian coronas do not contain a *new* radiation or *astral* substance; rather they are a **new order** induced on surrounding matter-energies under the biosystem's influence. PA-CO and external energies of DNAs are the most likely agents of these inductions.

The goal of *genetic biofeedback* is to detect PA-CO patterns of energy. It appears that at least a great part of Kirlian effects are due to PA-CO influence. Other effects superimposed on the Kirlian auras such as cellular, muscular, nerve or whatever physiological activities might cloud the characteristic inductive pattern of PA-CO shall be determined and neutralized or attenuated by carefully choosing experimental conditions.

Abundant data support the notion that coronas alter by emotions, mood, and above all, by **Will. Conscious Will** has been rated to be the most powerful stimulus affecting the corona, some subjects being able to make it appear and disappear altogether by **Will** alone. Is this not proof that **conscious Will** is the **integral-Will** of the system, and therefore able to control the whole system? A power so inclusive as to totally suppress induction of external orders, which implies complete control of the process of materializing internal energies.

The claims about *phantom images* are especially interesting. Mutilated portions of a leaf (up to 10% of the total area) appear in Kirlian photos although not with the intensity of the rest. Fingerprints of people who have lost the skin topography by burns and erosion are also revealed in Kirlian pictures. They appear as ghostly luminescence -indivisible by mechanical means!- with the peculiar patterns of the destroyed tissues. These are indisputable inductions of PA-CO, for the particular concrete cells reflected in *their phantom images* no longer exist.

The approximately 7,000 *acupuncture points* of Chinese tradition have been successfully located and validated by Kirlian techniques. They coincide with flares of singular brilliance in the auras. A very curious finding for surgical dissection never could trace them. Skin electrical resistance probing has been another successful procedure in the searching of acupuncture points and found such points in the same location given by the Kirlian effect.

In conclusion, Kirlian experimentation has showed that high frequency, high voltage electrical currents stimulates PA-CO and DNAs' external influences and facilitates the display of PA-CO energy orders. These orders differentiate themselves sufficiently (from the rest of physiological operations of a lower energetic

Maria L. Costell Gaydos

level) thus being considered potential candidates for *genetic biofeedback information*.

The biosystems' effects are not exclusively limited to the visual region of Kirlian photography, but might well embrace a wider spectrum of effects dependent on the surrounding media and stimuli of the biosystem.

In general, energetic patterns around biosystems, which are *not* produced exclusively by electromagnetic and non-biological energies, are potential sources for detection of external *genetic* orders. Additional screening procedures shall be studied to elucidate the effects of the two energetic levels: the *genetic* and the rest of the physiological activities.

Under the guidelines of this thesis the Kirlian work could be redefined, experimentation properly devised with diverse stimuli, and high frequency, high voltage biostimulation channeled to scientific endeavors. Since 1960 Russian Universities have been investigating the Kirlian phenomenon; however, they have not produced any theory to my knowledge that will account for bio-energies and programs of *genetic* self-regulation.

ENERGETIC PATTERNS OF HEALTHY AND CANCEROUS DNA.

The uncontrolled division of cancer cells reveals that cancerous DNA is apparently **isolated** from any social guidance and restrains. That is, the DNA's *energy* that in healthy cells is divided into *social* and *individual* functions, in cancer it is mostly used for the abnormal DNA's replication. This view is consistent with experimental facts. Cancer has been induced in healthy persons by inserting a sheet of plastic under subcutaneous tissue. **IF** the plastic was perforated cancer did *not* develop, suggesting that *not* the plastic itself but the **isolation** it creates from others cells was the cause of cancer. In other words, cancer is the lack of access to *social* interrelations with other cells, or in other cases, an access to *improper* PA-CO guidance.

The DNA's *social energy* is not only subtracted from the total DNA's energy, but it physically *disappears* engulfed in the energetic castle, which avidly converts *detectable* energy in the *non-detectable* types of energy and functions as thoughts, emotions, etc... Hence the individualistic cancerous DNAs, should render patterns of external energy *more intense* than those of healthy DNAs because their <u>unreleased</u> *social energy.* They have more energy to control external orders than do *social DNAs* for that purpose.

Arresting cancerous DNA division is an **off** process, a halting of action, that at the speed of DNA's reactions shall be *instantaneous.* The energetic change reflecting it should be abrupt and easily detectable. Such change would signal a re-programming of DNA responding to a re-programmed PA-CO energy under the command of the **Will**. The **Will's** control of DNAs or of PA-CO is carried out automatically via the castle of energies embodied in the body system. Biosystems can restore the proper functioning of their DNAs by **conscious Will**, because the built-in energy-controls are inescapable.

Thus, **Will** has the supreme role in using or misusing genetic resources. The *real cause* of *cancer* **is** a misuse of the **Will's** genetic control that most certainly would occur when the patient does not operate his **will** to produce healthy PA-CO patterns. Cancer will not appear if genetic control is rightly operated by the **Will**. The patients' **Will** shall be remembered, or taught again, how to handle the genetic complex.

Providing the **Will** with genetic feedback information gives the **Will** the opportunity to learn and to exercise adequate genetic control, and with it to cure cancer, AIDS and diseases tightly related to **genetic immunity**.

The spontaneous remissions of cancer tell us that the cure of cancer can be triggered by the patient himself, and the only way he could have done this is by stimulating his *genetic immunity*. The therapy to systematically reproduce spontaneous remissions of cancer is **Clinical Genetic Biofeedback**. For this it is needed to develop instrumentation that will feedback to the **conscious-Will** *instantaneous genetic information* (that is of PA-CO patterns) via *his PA-CO induced external orders.*

Research shall be aimed to develop said instruments to detect the changes of **PA-CO** patterns under the effect of the **Will.**

PA-CO can be reprogrammed at **Will** by *Genetic Biofeedback.* This is not only the only technique with theoretical foundations, as described by this theory, but medical literature also gives it overwhelming empirical support with its specific descriptions although unexplained findings of typically genetic diseases. We may add that there is **no other cure for cancer** because present treatments are in fact the destruction of cancer cells not the cure of them. The cure is the re-programming of their DNAs. Because DNA presides cellular activity, cancer remains in the body that has a cancerous PA-CO pattern, or its equivalent cancerous DNAs, and ready to burst out at the first opportunity.

GENETIC IMMUNITY AND AIDS.

We are under the impression that the nervous system is the ultimate animating principle of the body. The reality is quite different. To generate nerve activity, the stimuli should have a minimal strength, last long enough and reach minimal intensity. Only *then* will the responses turn on. This is plain evidence that any nerve action is a macro-effect of more elemental processes, those of the DNAs. This theory establishes that the

317

energy-castle of biosystems, subordinate to the **Will**, sets the states that trigger DNAs action, resulting in cellular action that eventually will translate into the body's action.

On this scheme of things, DNAs have the greatest energetic significance of the organism. First, from their intercommunications (external energies *within* the body) PA-CO and the energetic castle emerge. And second, out of their remaining energies (the internal energies of the DNAs), cellular activities are regulated. DNAs' energy level is *superior* to that of every material element of the body, otherwise no DNAs would preside cellular activity, which means all the body's actions.

Power, actual control, depends on informational content. It is the superb information of the DNA that makes it the most intelligent, receptive, and responsive molecule in the world. Its sensitivity, irritability, and speed of reaction are above cellular, nerve or any common physiological responses. These -that are activated by the **Will-** should first be channeled to the DNAs, to end finally in the cells of the nerve, muscular or any other system.

DNAs and not the nerve system are the concrete enervating principle of the body.

Let's briefly consider the case of AIDS. Alien organizations owe their power to the quality of their orders. More intelligent orders control less intelligent ones. We shall not lose sight of the fact that viruses - AIDS included - are DNA molecules of various complexities. Products developed by the pharmaceutical industry to combat AIDS do not have the informational content of the viruses, much less that of the castle of energies of a virus that is *evolved* naturally from *within.* There is no way to *artificially* evolve a similar castle of energies.

The virus battle shall be fought and won with DNAs molecules, and there is no reason for human DNAs to succumb under the AIDS attack, having more powerful organization, acting in their own territory (man's body) and being helped by the accumulated inductive control of the organism. Obviously AIDS will be the one to succumb under the proper genetic immune reaction.

The fact that DNA failed in the battle against AIDS is again proof of the **Will**'s misuse of genetic resources, and/or the failure of the **Will** to correct and convert PA-CO AIDS patterns into healthy PA-CO patterns. The **patient's Will** cannot learn or be activated to fight AIDS in absence of *instantaneous* genetic information. By Clinical Genetic Biofeedback genetic immunity can be awakened and take care of this devastating disease. And that again is conditional upon the development of instrumentation that will *instantaneously* signal PA-CO reaction to AIDS under the guidance of the **conscious Will**. Present techniques are not satisfactory in the treatment of AIDS, which has reached global epidemic proportions and keeps spreading at exponential rates. Time has become a critical factor not only to save the AIDS patients but to save the world population.

CONCLUSION: FUNDING SHALL BE DIRECTED TOWARDS CLINICAL GENETIC BIOFEEDBACK.

Cancer, AIDS and genetic disorders **urge the funding of development of instrumentation for Clinical Biofeedback at the genetic level.** PA-CO pattern changes respond to the command of the **conscious Will** while it directly guides the DNAs activities. The understanding and control of these changes by Genetic Biofeedback is of paramount importance, for it means conquering the **conscious control** of our genetic machinery.

At this time in History man has apparently lost the ability to wisely lead genetic defenses of self-protection. **Conscious Will** has corrupted its *inherent natural* goodness and strength leaving DNAs without any path to follow except its own, its DNAs codes of life. **Genetic Feedback instrumentation** is the absolutely needed **mirror** that will permit to restore genetic order to those patients afflicted with a chaotic genetic system. This approach will give men the tools to properly control a lethal enemy of unprecedented power, his unruled DNAs.

CHAPTER XIV. – GENETIC IMMUNITY, PHYSIOLOGICAL IMMUNITY.

ENERGETIC PATTERNS OF HEALTHY AND CANCEROUS DNAs.

The uncontrolled division of cancer cells reveals that cancerous DNA is apparently **isolated** from any social guidance and restrains normally governing the body. That implies that the DNAs' energy which in healthy cells is divided into *social* and *individual* functions, in cancer it is mostly used for abnormal DNA's replication.

Healthy DNA ought to have less *concrete* energy than a cancerous one because it relates energetically to other DNAs. The DNA's *social energy* in cancer patients is not only subtracted from the total DNA's energy, but it physically *disappears* engulfed in the energetic castle, which avidly converts *detectable* energy in the *non-*

detectable types of energy and functions as thoughts, emotions, etc., The energy of DNAs inter-relations generate the PA-CO matrix that evolves into superior energies instantaneously formed. Those energies up to the **Will** are progressively less detectable, and that means that the energetic contributions of healthy DNAs vanish from the *concrete* deducting such energy from the total DNAs' energy. Instead the cancerous DNA does not cooperate with the social enterprise, keeping its energy in the concrete world of physic-chemical reactions *instrumentally detectable*. Hence the *individualistic* cancerous DNAs should render external energetic orders *more intense* than those of healthy *social* DNAs due to their *unreleased social energy*. That is, they have *more energy to control external orders* than social DNAs have for that purpose. The same DNA *concrete* energetic superiority over body molecules results in the internal disorders of physiological functions in cancer patients. Cancer acts more like an invading virus than like a social component of the body, although the difference of both is crucial. Cancerous DNA *is* part of the body and might become normal again while the virus cannot and shall thus be destroyed by immunity resources.

The theory that cancer is caused by a virus has been abandoned about four decades ago by many empirical reasons. Cancerous tumors rarely contain any active virus, virus particles or antibodies that are produced as response to virus infection. None of these are found in any tumor that may have had millions of allegedly infected cells. Thus, if viruses caused cancer they would have left at least some traces or response to their prolific replications. In addition, it is characteristic of cancer, especially of cervical ones, to originate from one single cell that *continues living and dividing out of control.* Viruses on the other hand are the ones that replicate themselves *without control* in the infected cells using their resources and *causing their death* instead of their reproduction. Contrary to viral infection the immune system unfortunately does not recognize cancer cells as foreign to the body, which they certainly are not, and therefore does not fight them with antibodies or any other *physiological immune* reaction.

Arresting cancerous DNA division is an **off** process, a halting of action, which at the speed of DNA's reactions should be an *instantaneous* response to a re-established *healthy PA-CO energy.* The energetic change reflecting the correction of DNA and PA-CO energies should be an abrupt one easily *detectable in PA-CO induced external order.* I refer to *PA-CO induced external orders* because **that** is our target, the compiled DNAs' inter-communication relations, and the powerful pattern of energies that preside DNAs' activities. Such change would signal the re-programming of PA-CO, which will inevitably effect the re-programming of cancerous DNAs whatever their number would be. The **Will's** control of DNAs' energies or of PA-CO's energy is carried out automatically via the castle of energies embodied in the body system.

Biosystems may restore the proper functioning of their DNAs or compel their self repair mechanisms by **conscious Will,** because the built-in energy-controls are *inescapable* and admirably designed to convey the **Will'**s control of the body in general and of each of its minutest elements in particular. In this supreme role that **will** has to manipulate genetic resources can be found the cure of cancer, in fact, the cure of every disease as all of them have an *initial* genetic component.

Can **voluntary genetic control** be taught? Absolutely! A child just born does *not* know how to move his fingers. By looking at them the child is able to link **Will's decisions** with **fingers' moves**. He learns aided by feedback information: the vision of his fingers. Once he masters the voluntary control of them he somehow engraves this learning in his body to become a habitual control ever after with a minimum conscious effort. A concert pianist brings this learning ability to extraordinary levels of complexity and shall better describe such technique to the reader. But don't miss the point: the child has learned **to voluntarily control his DNAs** in relation to *his* fingers movement. The *voluntary* control of DNAs had resulted in the conscious *voluntary* movement and subsequent habitual reflexes of his fingers. The **Will** has been educated in using the well-coordinated link **Will-DNAs** to move the finger despite not knowing the reactions involved in such a specific task.

The same child, and by the same built-up power, can control the genetic complex in every other aspect, including cancer, providing that his **conscious Will** would receive proper genetic feedback information from the result of **its** decisions. For instance, it can be devised as feedback information a pleasant sound when the **Will** induces a healthy PA-CO. In contrast an unpleasant noise if the induced PA-CO is a cancerous one. This acoustic information that the child either will enjoy or will avoid gives his **Will** the opportunity to indirectly (by ear) learn and exercise adequate genetic control, to cure cancer. Moreover, to prevent it permanently as a reflex control! See in Chapter XII the conclusive experiments by Dr. Basmajian on the conscious and subconscious control of *one single* nerve-cell.

The spontaneous remissions of cancer tell us that the patient himself can trigger the cure of cancer, and the only way he could have done it, when medical treatment had been discontinued, is by stimulating his *genetic immunity*. That is, reprogramming his genetic machinery to the proper function to erase cancer. The therapy to systematically reproduce spontaneous remissions of cancer is only one: Clinical Genetic Biofeedback.

There is no theoretical possibility to reprogram cancer DNAs by *wired-in* processes. The whole body's structure works at once on each change and has the intelligence and power to perform it at the command of the **Will**. PA-CO, the presiding guidance of DNAs, can be reprogrammed at **Will** by *Genetic Biofeedback*. For this it is urgently needed to develop instrumentation that will feedback to the **conscious-Will** *instantaneous genetic information* (about PA-CO healthy or not healthy patterns) using *the PA-CO induced external orders*. This is not only the way to reach the *real cure of cancer* based on a theoretical foundation, as described by this theory, but it is the **safest, quickest and most precise treatment** to be found: the one devised by the biosystem itself throughout eons of evolutionary improvements! *Safest*, for no external system intrudes the body or interferes with the body's functions. *Quickest*, for the reprogramming is done almost instantaneously at the speed of the castle of energies, which we assume to be faster than light. And more *precise* than any *wired-in* intervention incapable to localize and repair the genetic culprit. We may add that there is **no other possible cure for cancer** because external agents do not have the intelligence and power that the biosystem has for its own governing.

Present treatments are nothing other than the destruction of cancer cells by surgery, radiation or chemicals opposed to the *cure* of them and; on the way, killing healthy cells too. Medical treatments are barely cleaning or destroying the abnormalities that cancer is incessantly producing. These treatments maim the body and stop the growth of cells needed to replace tissues thus causing hair loss, anemia, muscle waste and depletion of physiological immune resources. The so-called *gene* therapies are based on the same principle, stimulate the *physiological immune system* in order to recognize and kill gene-modified cancerous cells. This is not correction of the *genetic* operation of DNAs or of PA-CO. It is a killing at the *physiological level* as such is the level of killed-cells and killing-cells. And because DNA presides cellular activity, cancer remains in *that* body that has *cancerous* DNAs, or the equivalent a *cancerous* PA-CO pattern, thus ready to burst out in any other location at the first opportunity.

The cure of cancer rests is the re-programming of PA-CO cancerous programs to healthy ones by **Will** and the new programs will induce the cure of cancerous DNAs and the repair of damaged DNAs. That is, the **Will** will stimulate **genetic immunity** where it resides, in the DNAs.

After more than half a century of medical failures and billions of dollars in failed avenues we must turn to this new treatment of Clinical Genetic Feedback.

THE CURE OF AIDS.

The bodies of living creatures respond to attack or injury by an immunity response either at the physiological level or at the genetic level. Medical and biological knowledge, giving the current principles of physics, doesn't go beyond the physiological level. It is self evident that diseases immediately related to **genetic material**, as cancer and AIDS, logically shall be repelled by an immune reaction at the **genetic** level. As soon as we accept this fact the sooner **cancer** and **AIDS** will be cured.

Let's briefly review the history of AIDS.

AIDS, for Acquired Immune Deficiency Syndrome, has been defined as a deficiency of the *physiological immunity system* that disable it to fight well known infections. There are no particular or unique combinations of diseases that are *exclusive* of AIDS. Certain patients may develop altogether different ones than other patients. Thus a list of them, that grows every year, has been compiled to help doctors diagnose AIDS patients. These are called "opportunistic infections" and although they are due to diverse causes, in the case of AIDS patients the common denominator is the inability of the physiological immune system to cope with them. The active immune agents, T-cells, have been reduced to a fatally low number.

Pneumonias, cancers as Kaposi's sarcoma, cervical cancer, several lymphomas, herpes and yeast infections, syphilis, tuberculosis, and about thirty other diseases are counted today as members of the AIDS syndrome. Different types of infections than those common among Americans afflict African AIDS patients. Hemophiliacs who contract AIDS by blood transfusion, also develop infections of their own unrelated to the ones carried by the blood source.

The first symptoms of AIDS are similar to those of flu or mononucleosis. In one or two weeks they are aggravated by fever, fatigue, headache, sore throat, nausea, vomiting, muscle pain, loss of weight. In time the condition worsen to severe infections, uncontrollable, chronic diarrhea, lung and muscle waste and dementia from brain degeneration. A slow, sure and painful death!

Since 1985 the vast medical consensus has been established that AIDS is produced by the retrovirus HIV, human immunodeficiency virus, which presents itself in two forms HIV-1 and HIV-2. The last one most commonly found in African countries. Controversy and strong dissent about this theory abound to the point of allegations of malpractice, fraud investigations and lawsuits that do not concern us in our present work.

Viruses are *not living* micro-organisms composed of genetic molecules (DNA or RNA) that invade cells to produce many identical virus. They need the resources of the host cell they infect to grow and replicate, at times millions of them, causing the cell's death. The body reacts to viruses by producing specific antibodies that eliminate them. Antibiotics kill bacteria, a living micro-organism far more complex than viruses and easier to be recognized, but are useless against viruses. Viral infections instead are treated with vaccines. These inactivated or weakened forms of the virus stimulate the production of antibodies that eventually will clear up the virus from the system. But there are no vaccines either against HIV or AIDS. It is accepted that once HIV invades the body the immune system is doomed to collapse, and what is worse, and absolutely true under current medical *wired-in* theories, *there is no possible cure.* Apparently HIV remains in a latent state ready to keep reproducing and killing T-cells while life lasts. The AIDS patient is left defenseless against any disease that otherwise is treatable and cured in non-HIV-infected people. With the *physiological immune system* devastated the whole body is eaten away even by innocuous microbes that the body hosts. Hundreds of them which did not previously give any problem! Pneumonia is a good example of disease due to such microorganisms that become active when the immune system deteriorates by chemotherapy treatments.

Contrary to other viruses HIV who disappeared under the attack of antibodies, HIV is not considered to have been cleared up, and the presence of specific HIV antibodies is precisely the main factor in the diagnosis of AIDS. Patients of a garden variety of infections become officially AIDS patients: 1) when HIV antibodies are found *despite that the actual HIV may not be detected,* and 2) when T-cells -the active agents of the immune system- are less than 200 per ml. of blood. The normal T-cells level is between 450 to 1,200 per ml.

Thus, the AIDS diagnosis shall be made by a medical doctor *after considering* a combination of factors: T-cell counting, HIV testing and symptoms of some *listed* AIDS' opportunistic diseases.

The first case of AIDS was diagnosed in 1980 to reach more than one million HIV positive tested cases by the next decade. Presently the world population has about 1.35 billion HIV positive tested of which 22.8 million are in United States. Russians recently reported 1.5 million. Africa counts 30 million with 5.3 million in South Africa. Of the American HIV positive tested only 1/3 developed AIDS after a decade. This prompted experts to extent the *latent* incubation period for the virus to more than 10 years. The other 2/3 then are expectant AIDS patients.

AIDS is mainly confined to certain "group risks" out of which the percentage of cases is far less. Based on this statistic some biologists claim that AIDS is not contagious. At least no more contagious than the particular infection would be in non-AIDS patients. But while *viral diseases are not a death sentence,* AIDS sure is. Frequent AIDS victims are drug and alcohol abusers, people engaged in promiscuous sexual activity, or with a long history of venereal diseases, homosexuals, especially those with repeated hepatitis B, and children born from mothers with AIDS, a history of drug addiction or chronic venereal diseases. A study in South Carolina describes "trauma" to be one of the causes of AIDS in children. The report points to 34% having a parent habitually drunk and 25% having suffered sexual abuse. Hemophiliacs are especially vulnerable to AIDS for they depend on blood transfusions that may be contaminated, plus, blood transfusions themselves are immunosuppressive.

There is no surprise about these "risk groups" being the targets of AIDS because to start with, *drugs' toxicity devastates the immune system.* Most nitrites used as recreational drugs, sodium alkyl or alkylated, when mixed with water produce nitrous acid which destroy all biological molecules. Drug users regularly lose white blood cells, the cornerstone of the immune system. Cocaine suppresses growth of T-cells. We may add to the problem the continuous abuse of antibiotics also immunosuppressive, malnutrition, protein and vitamin deficiency that plague these groups in their struggle to fight infections and to finance drug habits. Over a period of years the damage to the immune system is beyond repair. Some AIDS patients were never infected with HIV, the drugs took care of sweeping out their immune system.

There are no answers to many questions of the AIDS puzzle, why nine in ten AIDS patients in America are men or that in some African tribes only women get AIDS, that some AIDS patients have been tested HIV negative, or that a great number of HIV positive people do not develop AIDS at all, that no virus particles or very few are found in AIDS patients blood or tumors while in every viral infection -as hepatitis B- a few drops of blood renders about ten million of them, or why normal virus infections develop almost immediately but in the case of HIV it requires an incubation period of ten or more years. Obviously the *genetic material* has its own mysteries.

In 1970 the reverse transcriptase was discovered, an enzyme that explains how retroviruses work. A retrovirus copies the virus' genetic information from its RNA into cell's DNA, the *reverse* of the cell's process in which DNA presides the formation of RNA. This new RNA copy integrates into the genetic structure of the infected cell sealing its deadly fate.

In 1984 the discovery of the retrovirus HIV as the *AIDS virus* was announced, and ever since this view, overpowering or disregarding opposition has been the prevalent one. Rapidly the federal government and private institutions took unprecedent steps. Condoms and sterile needles were freely provided, even by Churches, to control the dissemination of the *highly communicable* AIDS.

In 1987 AZT (azidithymide) also known as Zidovudine or Retrovir was also announced in US as treatment for AIDS. It was followed by ddI (didanosine), ddC (zalcitabine) and others nucleoside reverse transcriptase inhibitors, better known as "nukes", *none of which cures AIDS*. This group of drugs, and the "non-nukes" for non nucleoside reverse transcriptase inhibitors, block in different ways the process by which HIV converts its RNA into DNA. That is, the drugs attempt although *none cure AIDS*. Actually these drugs obstruct cell division, they are extremely toxic and their side effects exacerbates the depletion of the physiological immune system. As cancer patients in chemotherapy treatments, AIDS patients treated with AZT develop anemia, loss of hair, waste of muscles and lymphoma. Most stricken yet because these symptoms appeared in HIV positive people that were treated in preventive basis with AZT *before* having any symptoms. By 1993 studies on 2,000 cases reported that *life* has not even been extended on those patients under AZT treatment. The cost to cope with AIDS is staggering. More than **22 billion** dollars were spent by 1994.

The most recent groups of drugs approved by the FDA are the protease inhibitors and immune stimulators. The problem with them is that they do not have the capability to *reprogram* inefficient or genetic defective DNAs nor to *recognize* which DNAs shall be reprogrammed to stimulate *genetic* immunity, which will translate into *physiological* immunity. A step sine qua non because *cellular* processes are induced by *genetic* ones! The drug's lack of knowledge about *what to do* is just the same lack of knowledge biologists and the rest of us have about the DNAs of other creatures. Despite having –all of us, at all times– the total command of *every single DNA of our systems* as Dr. Basmajian so demonstrated. Like every biosystem has! Without such knowledge, no drug can be intelligently planned to cure AIDS.

Therefore let's turn to the real possibilities of an **AIDS cure.**

Systems' organizations owe their power to the quality of their orders. More intelligent systems, structures or orders control less intelligent ones. We shall not lose sight of the fact that viruses –AIDS included – are DNA or RNA molecules of various complexities. Products developed by the pharmaceutical industry to combat AIDS do not have the informational content of viruses, much less that of the castle of energies of a virus that is *evolved* naturally from *within*. It is impossible to evolve a similar castle of energies *artificially*. Let's not even begin to enter into the complexities of human DNA and human castle of energy.

The virus battle shall be fought and won at the *genetic* level between human DNAs molecules and viruses' DNAs and RNAs. There is no reason for human DNAs to succumb under the AIDS attack having more powerful organization, acting in their own territory (man's body) and being helped by the accumulated inductive control of the organism. Obviously AIDS viruses should be the one to succumb under the proper DNAs' genetic immune reaction.

Should AIDS not be produced by a virus, let the human DNAs figured out the proper *genetic immune* reaction to the cause of AIDS whatever it may be.

That DNA failed in the battle against AIDS is nothing other than the **Will**'s misuse of genetic resources, the failure of the **Will** to convert **PA-CO-AIDS** patterns into healthy PA-CO patterns. The first ones betray the body's system allowing the virus' invasion. The second ones should combat the viruses with **genetic** immune resources better than any vaccine can by triggering **physiological** immune reactions. The reason is clear. Genetic reactions are energetically superior in quantity and quality to the physiological ones.

Genetic immunity can be awakened and will take care of this devastating disease by **Clinical Genetic Biofeedback.** This treatment requires the development

337

of instrumentation that will *instantaneously signal* PA-CO *induced external orders*. A person must receive *instantaneous* genetic information to learn how to **directly** manipulate or control his genetic mechanisms because the communication between **Will** and PA-CO is practically *instantaneous.* Any delay would make meaningless to the subject the effect of his **Will** upon a **genetic** reaction.

The problems to solve for the development of such instrumentation are two: 1) to detect specifically the *PA-CO induced external orders* on matter-energy, and 2) to translate the changes of such orders into almost *instantaneous signals* -sounds, graphs.,etc- which the subject may interpret as resulting from his **Will.**

Calibration of the instrumentation will depend on **the specific genetic control to be mastered.** With two groups of AIDS patients and healthy people can be obtained the signals given by each group. The AIDS patient shall be trained to match the healthy signals by **Will** or aided by mental programs. With time, as a child or a pianist master DNAs to move their fingers, he will activate habitually his DNAs against AIDS. The same instrument may be calibrated for other diseases with groups of cancer patients, diabetics, or the long list of patients with unsolved diseases. The patients will learn to activate by **conscious Will** the genetic immunity against these diseases. Clinical Genetic Feedback offers a direct, clean, efficient control of the **Will** upon DNAs and DNAs defense of the body!

CONCLUSION: THE URGENCY TO DEVELOP GENETIC FEEDBACK INSTRUMENTATION.

Present medical approaches are not satisfactory in the treatment of **cancer** or **AIDS,** which have reached global epidemic proportions and keep spreading at alarming rates. Time has become a critical factor, not just to save the AIDS patients but to save the world population. The DNAs' system of these patients is practically destroyed because we have not yet developed the skill to *govern our genes* by **conscious Will.** And precisely when they are under attack, they are the sole *competent* army against those adversaries. In the case of cancer, DNAs have abandoned their social behavior and are left without any path to follow except its own codes of life. These now, in an unruled body, dictate individualistic, erratic and unstopping reproduction. In the case of AIDS the physiological immune system has collapsed because the viruses have lured or tricked the DNAs into their service. A fatal degeneration and disintegration of the body! Superior organizations degraded to inferior functions.

Conscious Will has an *inherent natural* intelligence and power to wisely mobilize genetic defenses to protect the body. PA-CO pattern of energies respond to the command of the **conscious Will** and PA-CO guides directly the DNAs activities. The understanding and control of PA-CO by Genetic Biofeedback is of paramount importance, for it means conquering the **conscious control** of the genetic machinery and winning the genetic battles against a genetic system in disarray.

Theory and empirical precedents for **Clinical Genetic Biofeedback** have been exposed in this thesis. It has been abundantly proven, for no money or efforts had been spared, that present avenues towards the cure of **Cancer, AIDS and genetic diseases have failed.** At this time in History not to learn voluntary genetic control will lead to the actual extermination of man. A share of government and private efforts and funding need to be invested in the development of **Genetic Feedback Instrumentation,** absolutely needed to restore order in chaotic genetic systems.

CHAPTER XV. – SYSTEMS ARE CONCRETE INFORMATIOM AND ABSTRACT IDENTITIES.

This theory was initially named the "Theory of Physical Reality" and later changed to the "Theory of Systems" because all physical reality sensorially perceived or instrumentally detected is a system and it is *concrete* information. The most elemental matter-energy cannot be known for there are insurmountable barriers to empirical knowledge of *the elemental physical reality* as Heisenberg discovered.

In our inquiry on systems we have discussed the *transferable,* detectable reality, the *concrete* that we termed *information*, and the *non transferable,* essential and inherently born with the system – as it is *its identity- whose nature is known by its effects*. **Identity** of the being is an *abstraction* that escapes instrumental detection.

This thesis found throughout rationalization that there are two fundamental *abstract faculties* essential to each identity: a) *intelligence*, the capability to draw meaning from information, *and* b) *freedom to decide,* the capability to chose between alternatives. (I left out *social drive* for later). By mental elimination we may reach *what* can be reduced to be the *most elemental intelligence:* the awareness of self as distinct from non-self, and *what* can be *the most elemental freedom to decide:* to act or not to act. These are the *abstract* faculties of the *ultimate physical reality,* whose *concrete* aspects cannot be known by Physics, nor by any other discipline, not because deficiencies on the instrumentation but because the *nature of concrete reality* itself. The theory of systems, by incorporating *the abstract* in the probe of reality, goes beyond present scientific limits.

The significance of *the abstract* is its governing power over *the concrete* through intelligence, will, and ultimately action from within the *identity* rather than from outside of it. In this sense, *physical reality* is primarily an **abstraction**, an **order** imposed upon a number of components. The *abstract* determines life and death in animate beings, and the very existence of the inanimate ones.

ABSTRACT REALITIES.

We are the witnesses and agents within our own beings not only of the existence of *the abstract* but also of the processes of abstraction and dematerialization. We materialize *ideas* into concrete creations, and conversely, sensing material beings we elevate them to images and later to *ideas*, the sublimation where no form abides.

For too long, it has been retained that *the abstract* and *the process of abstraction* are the exclusive prerogative of man. That implies that man is made up of substances imported from beyond the Creation. Can a scientist accept this implication? If not, abstraction and the process of abstraction should be investigated here within *physical reality,* better renamed it simply **reality**. Science has already taken steps in this direction. Einstein's stroke of equalizing matter and energy was a sort of dematerialization of matter.

Atomic bonding are classified under two denominations: *localized* and *de-localized* or in **resonance**. The atoms in benzene are linked by *de-localized* ones and its structure is symbolized by two formulas attempting to best express the *inexpressible in concrete dimensions*, for those bonds, or their interconversion, already transcend *concrete* reality. The real benzene molecule fluctuates between the properties represented by graphics

343

1 and 2, an hexagonal structural arrangement of atoms each having the double bonds in different locations, without trace of intermediate states.

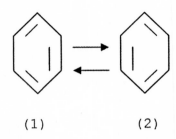

(1)   (2)

If light is said to have the properties of *wave* and *particle*, though nobody went so far as to say, <u>simultaneously</u>, *then a transformation process is at work!* Neither did anybody set the speed of conversion from one form to the other. The same *duality* has been applied to electrons, elemental particles, and matter in general. A wave is associated to matter. These descriptions are accepted today as *scientific* despite that they are indeed *irreconcilable* and inadmissible on physical dimensions, and without theoretical basis, such notions are but concessions that defeat reason and logic, which are the sole intellectual tools of Physics.

A legitimate avenue to revive validity to scientific thought is to include in the *concept of reality* the essential attributes of identity, intelligence, freedom, social drives and the faculty to perform dematerialization processes up to pure abstraction.

Moreover, when mathematical abstraction is the base of science, abstraction has been accepted to be evident, and the effects of *the abstract* are palpable realities that could only emanate from it. The study of *reality* cannot subsist much longer ignoring the abstract and the ascending dematerialization of energies without becoming an intellectual undertaking with no significant future.

This thesis offers the new concept of **control-energies** evolving from association of energetic elements by and with increasing quantitative and qualitative informational content. Each succeeding evolvement represents *new orders, new dimensions* whose capacities exceed the preceding dimension from where they came. Image's dimensions do not represent every flower that might have been or will be created. It is the *idea* that embraces them all in one single and more capable dimension. It is evident that when information increases it forces the creation of a more dematerialized pattern (so to say), which constitutes another less materialized dimension. Holograms, virtual images on mirrors, give us a *taste* of the process of dematerialization.

But there is more. Physical reality cannot exist, or biosystems survive, without the power of *abstraction.* How can the reader recognize what plants, animals, or men are, if he is only capable of retaining and storing the *specifics* of each particular entity? How it is possible to find or to apply the *law* without the *idea of the law*? How do animals avert danger and search for food and shelter in a world where *past experiences* never repeat themselves identically? Add to the list the prophetic vision that gear purpose and action to unfold evolution and you will have ample support for the need of *the abstract.*

All *life* has the faculty *to abstract* in order to exist and to survive. The feelings of fear, joy, love, etc., are undeniable *abstract* energies. They are manifested in some degree in the lowest organisms. They imply the recognition of the self, and transcend *to the recognition of their species.* In superior organisms abstract capabilities have further evolved. Man's abstract power reaches the frontiers of the universe, the unseen, the gone, and the highest abstraction: God, for the human mind by some mysterious intuition has been able to probe this highest of levels. The *intangibles* are common to all *life.*

This thesis extends abstract faculties *to all reality* and categorically rejects any distinction whatsoever among the substantial **essences** of the Creation. Differences of these faculties among its creatures arise from *the different levels of evolvement of orders*, not for the importation of them from out of the universe. The raw material of physical reality is one and the same from the Big Bang to our present day. *Freedom*

346

and *intelligence* are inalienable essences of universal reality and the presiding controls of the concrete.

Starting at the most elemental level *freedom and intelligence* are *essential* ingredients of reality, one requiring the other. To have intelligence without freedom would yield *perfect order* where no freedom of man or beast would abide. With no intelligence to process information nothing would in fact be useful. Information not only would be a waste, but systems (if they ever emerge by some miracle) would be locked in sheer isolation. Therefore, evolution would be absolutely unable to proceed. The universe would be one inhabited by data encapsulated in their own impenetrable shield, physical dimension inscrutable by comprehension. No orders would have been developed after the Big Bang. What did I say? The Big Bang would not have occurred for its cause was primarily communication among physical realities.

The Bell's Theorem demonstrated that *isolation* and *quantum principles* are incompatible. One of these propositions **is** false. The theory of systems retains both notions to be false because isolation and quantum principles are partial visions of reality. No sketch of the universe that segregates a part of it is valid as a general theory for its interpretation. Reality is integrated by the concrete and the abstract, and those previous notions address only one segment of reality.

347

These preliminaries show that any opposition to the postulates of the theory of systems actually is (when logically scrutinized) unacceptable to science, to reason, to feelings and to empirical observation. **Wills** to decide action, or freedom of decision, and **intelligence** to draw meaning from information, are *essential* to reality, absolutely needed by the concrete world and generating its very existence as described by this theory.

REALITIES AND DIMENSIONS.

Systems, that is, information, provide the material for drawing *meaning* and the build-in *controlling power* of energy. Both *control-energy* and *intelligence* rigorously fit informational-content when considering its quantitative and qualitative aspects.

I cannot conceive that any system, man included, might have any other type of intelligence than the automatic faculty to interpret its informational content. The use of the interpretation is another story! That is the prerogative of the freedom to decide. I do not see any difference between intelligence and knowledge (that is, *information* already processed, from which *meaning* has been derived) save the conceptual one assigning to the first the role of *container, processor, agent,* leaving to the second the role of *content, processed, meaning.*

Why should drifty Nature provide bigger dimensions or bigger containers (or varied ones) than the stuff they contain? Are such containers necessary? If it happens to be so, the next question is rushing behind: *Under what standards are such extravagant, oversized packagings manufactured?* The contrary proposition *"for matter-energy to have less intelligent capability than the information contained for processing, or no capacity at all"* (as Physics stands presently for the inanimate), **is** precisely what the theory of systems is **contesting**. That is, that the *concrete* is devoid of the *abstract*. The postulate of the theory of systems as they relate to the above mentioned can be stated in these terms: **"There are no dimensions apart from reality"**.

Association of matter-energy -and no other dimensions- creates information, systems, reality. **Free Wills** or control-energies are *narrowed* to the energies they control; they are *specific* and *exclusive* to each energy-control. **Free Will** entails limited decisions. No **cellular-will** can decide for an organ or a system, its decisions are strictly *cellular* in regard to the *specific cell* it governs and no other. Likewise **intelligence** to draw meanings out of information are supported and *limited to such information*. Hence inanimate beings, plants and man, differ in their quantitative and qualitative degree of freedom, which may be assessed in terms of information. Nevertheless the **freedom** of man

349

is grounded and justified in the **freedom** of all reality and in its process of evolvement.

Energy-control and *intelligence* are automatically created by association of information or systems and **there is no other dimensions in the universe than the systems and their faculties.**

FREEDOM IS THE ULTIMATE VARIABLE OF REALITY. ASSOCIATION IS THE SOLE TOOL OF CREATION OR EVOLUTION.

Freedom is the ultimate variable of reality. Neither meaning, nor information are *variables* for they depend on other realities. Intelligence is a *function* of information but free decision is totally independent. It has the absolute power to decide and to decide *unintelligently* if it pleases. Information, instead, is a fact, a finished pattern. *Meaning* is inflexible, it is one and ever the same upon a given information. This inflexibility is the basis of the notion of **truth.**

Free Will may adopt two opposite positions in front of a *unique* meaning for it is **free.** *It might create two different realities.* By **Will**'s action one reality out of two possibilities becomes a new system, a new **identity** with a new **Will.** Creation of a system is always *spontaneous* creation of new interrelations, new qualities unrelated to the previous ones, new intelligences, new wills, therefore new identities. **Wills** do not travel, are not transferable. They are *created* **free** as the unpredictability of the system attests. **This is a creation. This is evolution.**

The core of evolution is association, not randomly done, but actualizing harmonic relationships among associates. This kind of enterprise requires *freedom* and *intelligence*. Without the first the universe would plunge into a deterministic harmonic utopia; without the second the universe would be a pool of chaotic associations, if any ever would result; without both only a universe of *synthetic intelligence* is possible providing that a *natural intelligence* resides beyond its limits working incessantly *synthesizing* it. Thus, the **identity** of each system directly relates to its **Will** and **intelligence** compounded, for one cannot exist without the other.

Evolution requires a *drive to associate* that is obviously part and parcel of reality. For while it is true that there is elemental matter *unassociated* in the interstellar spaces, this same elemental matter is found to be *associated* in almost every system. The drive of association is there but its use on care of the free will has taken different paths.

The theory of systems rejects the quantum theory doctrine that required an *observer* to collapse the possibilities of the Schödinger equation into *realities*.

Why should there be an *outside observer* needed when each free-intelligent reality *is the observer* of its own being? Or rather how is an *observer* able to observe the *outside reality* but cannot observe *itself*? What the quantum interpretation does not punctuate is *where* and *when* the observation should be made, *what* should be observed when *that reality is still non-existent? What type of observer* would cause the collapse into *reality*? A man, a rabbit, an atom? In absence of these determinants the theory of systems does not find objection to locate, to time and to equate **the observer** with **the reality itself** in the act of **self-awareness. Reality** that acts by feedback information along the entire universe certainly is *aware of its own self,* because it must recognize <u>the aim of its **Will**</u> in order to get the wanted results. To recognize **Will**'s *aim* implies recognizing <u>*its* **Will**</u>, *the integral control of its system, in other words, its* <u>*soul*</u>, *for such is the* <u>*animating force*</u> *of the system.*

Let us not betray the facts. The universe collapsed before man could observe it because a preliminary universe is needed to evolve man.

GENERALIZATION OF THE THEORY OF SYSTEMS.

Elements that generate systems are not to be necessarily material ones. Being matter-energy interchangeable, systems may also spring merely from energies. The energetic castle of biosystems in itself is a system. It has *intelligence* and indeed has **free Will** that we identify with a familiar name, the **soul** of the identity.

"Any consolidated physical energies, two or more, during a time interval of union, or any energetic aspect, whatsoever of reality is a system and a subsystem of the universe."

When an order is established, new qualities appear that belong solely to *that* order. For example, frequently products *spontaneously associated* might join their effects into a more active or energetic result than the calculated sum of their effects acting alone. This phenomenon is called *synergism* and should be understood as the *expression of new control-energies* evolved in the association. Or what is very common, new marvels appear that surpass expectations. An amorph substance is a barrier to the light that freely crosses the same substance when setup into an *ordered* crystal. In general the gathering of individual resources renders advantages to the collectivity.

Through natural association there is a growth of order and harmony in the *concrete*, intelligence and wills in the *abstract,* and a sequence of intertransformable *energy-controls* that connects both. The new *identity* is inherently attached to the associated information, that is, to reality. And its uniquely built-in energy-controls that transcend to the exterior inducing order and harmony.

The life of a system may vary from the temporal as seasonal migration of birds, herds or mating habits, to the permanent colonies of insects that last the long life of the queen and out of which no individual survives. The longest lasting system, the universe, counts an age of about 20 billion years and could go on a few hundred billion more.

The theory of systems refers only to the natural systems for this is critically important to differentiate *natural* from *artificial* ones. The first are *spontaneously* created, *inherently* intelligent and free, and *identifiable by their effects and their capabilities of control.* The second ones are barely tools to process and match information. There are not *intelligences* to interpret and judge information and **wills** to freely decide even to the point of wrongly decidinge upon correct information. Listed in this second type are the synthetic intelligences (instruments, computers, robots, etc) and the social, economical and cultural structures.

It is impossible to dissect a *natural system*, as it is the usual analytic method of science. Systems should be evaluated qualitatively instead of quantitatively because in their *identities* and *functions* are based the significance of their *unique orders,* not in the weight and measure of their components. Nor is it possible to evaluate natural systems by the number of its interrelations for this is not measurable either and most interrelations depart from the concrete. This uniqueness becomes more obvious with the increasing complexity of the systems. Thus, systems are more *orders* than *things* and ought to be studied and handled on their own terms: orders, patterns, energy-controls and creative decisions. Laws are not imposed upon them. Systems make their own laws, which are no more than *descriptions of their activity.* Their **freedom** is absolute. Systems are not evolutionary accidents. They decide their associations and evolvements. They are evolution itself.

These are some of the characters of *natural systems* that constitute all reality of the Creation.

Maria L. Costell Gaydos

COMMUNICATION OF INFORMATION AND KNOWLEDGE.

We are familiar with established concepts of communication via matter-energy transfer and reactions, the maximum speed being that of light. But if there is communication between the abstract by force such communication must be conducted on abstract dimensions, which may well exceed light speed, for the abstract to dominate the concrete dimensions. A change of pattern *instantaneously* affects the *whole* pattern. Comprehension of the abstract is comprehension of the *whole*, which is indivisible and does not admit chained reasoning or apprehension by sections. It should be understood all *at once*, although the intelligent agent may need preparation time to develop the fitness for the task.

Abstraction as *a process comes to solve the incapability of the physical world to indefinitely absorb information*, that is, *concrete* items. With the idea **man** the mind accommodates every individual of the human race, with the idea **law** the mind embraces a general range of events. The particular material realities or events embraced by said ideas would occupy immense space and time when spelled in physical dimensions.

Empirical sciences lean too heavily on the *concrete* aspect of reality. Paradoxically Nature has solved precisely the *excess* of the concrete in the very substance of the abstract. As matter and energy can be transformed in each other, so the concrete and the abstract are interconvertible and part of each other. The accumulation of information obliges the progressive unshelling of the accidental that hides the abstract essences. It is this increase of information that makes *intelligences* and *wills* to be more patent in more complex creatures till they unmistakable are fully manifested in living beings.

The process of dematerialization is internally experienced in the course of sensorial print, image, and idea. While intelligence to draw meaning and **Will** to decide materialize on action following the opposite course. Back and forth materialization-dematerialization are universal processes in simple or in complex realities.

When leaving behind the *concrete* to enter the *non-tangible* concrete measurements ought to be left with the concrete. Still the abstract is firmly related to information. Dematerialization is designed to absorb and store excessive information. Materialization is required to utilize and communicate it.

Within the system small *intelligences* cannot apprehend the meaning of patterns entrusted to larger ones, and, as every system and subsystem are free, superior controls cannot take away the freedom of inferior ones. Such *trust* within the system transcends *concrete* information and its speed exceeds that of the concrete. The decider's faith that its decisions will be carried out instantaneously and almost blindly within the system is at the root of universal feedback self-regulation. I said *almost blindly* because nothing is absolutely certain among free realities except their freedom.

Chronologically, our universe operated entirely at the speed of light just a fraction of a second -around the Big Bang- it took to rise from the chaotic disorder. As soon as two energetic elements associated the **energy-control** bonding them, opened the door to faster than light speeds, the new avenues of communication of the abstract. *Control of the concrete* due to the increased informational-content started right there and **control-energies** grew in number and complexity parallel to the evolvement of orders. Information congregated into abstract patterns of greater complexity. And thus the universe enriched its orders, their *intelligence* and their ***Wills***. The *abstract* took over the *concrete* for all practical purposes and communication on the abstract level should have necessarily been faster than that on the concrete to overcome it.

Intellectual advancement is the only possible direction of an *informational* universe and this took place in the form of evolution. All elements of the creation have the same age, but evolutionary advancement was not uniform for every system. From the numerous paths that evolution took in its free choices, the one that resulted in the production of man was the most successful and speediest one. Man has more information and dimensions than any known system. He is the most eloquent piece of the universe's hologram and where *physical reality* shall be studied on its two aspects, *concrete* and *abstract*.

CHAPTER XVI. - CONFIRMATION OF THE THEORY OF SYSTEMS. WILL AND PHYSIOLOGICAL CONTROL.

Overwhelming empirical data attest the theory of systems, its principles and consequences. We shall not delay its practical medical applications.

Systems' intelligences and energy-controls are supremely adapted to *each* particular system. If that were not the case, a more qualified system would operate a *foreign* inferior one without any kind of trouble. Man would know perfectly, in a manner of speaking, the constitution and roles performed by an amoeba, a bird, a human DNA, and his own DNAs! To our regret this is not the real situation. Each system, or subsystem, zealously guards its own identity and related abstract faculties. The speedy game of photons, the reactions of the DNA, rating one million to a hundred million reactions per second, are being painfully deciphered at tremendous cost of work and money. In the favorable case that one-day, all possible *concrete* information of one biosystem will be piled up, we will still be short of knowing the self-**intelligence** and of possessing the self-**Will** of the system. Every system and subsystem is independent and has its own **Will**. Thus man's **conscious Will** merely *induces* its decisions to the DNAs of his body, which in turn accept them when such decisions are in harmony with their codes of life. DNA has its own intelligence, its own **Will**. There is no possible interchange of actors or supplanting *identities* in the theater of Nature for the universe is not a world of fantasy; *it is the real thing* which does not admit substitution.

The basic relation between **Will** and *physiological results* is totally proven. **Will** masters each and every body action and can correct errors of which it receives information.

In the case of hypnosis **Will**'s control is exercised despite the fact that the hypnotized subject has relinquished his **conscious Will** to that of the hypnotist.

For more than three decades surgeon Dr. Angel Escudero[4] is practicing surgery without chemical anesthesia. Pain is controlled by **Will**. **Will** dominates the intricate nerves' mechanisms of pain. Quoting Dr. Escudero's own words oF this technique he calls Noesitherapy: "The volitive psychoanalgesia (VPA) is programmed with only one *thought*, bringing into focus the idea of possession of the *desired* psychoanalgesia. - The patient obtains VPA by affirming that he has achieved it *in the area of the body where he needs it*, or in the whole body. And then the duration is programmed: hour, days, or until the wounds are cured."

Psychoanalgesia is therefore *locally specific* as elegantly demonstrated by Dr. Basmajian's experiments of single-cell control. But Noesitherapy goes further in two relevant aspects: 1) that the programming is done *days before* the surgery will take place, and 2) that the programming includes the *timing* and *duration* of the psychoanalgesia.[5] These last two interesting aspects of Noesitherapy unveils further capabilities of the **Will's control** and potential for habituation of healthy or unhealthy states.

Many studies to ascertain psychological influences in the occurrence of cancer show that the cancer patient exhibits a rigidity of **Will** and an *excess* of self-control strongly rationalized by a self-defeating idealism that restricts the adaptation response. It equates to lack of faith in the universal wisdom, a calling for death. DNA, a *code of life,* cannot accept it, nor will stop its natural activities. Energy will unlikely halt acting. On the other extreme it can be cited the edifying case of Dr. Hans Selye, famous worldwide for his studies in the general adaptation syndrome. He was diagnosed with incurable cancer giving no more than one year to live. After three years he was in complete remission, no trace of cancer left. He publicly declared: *"I beat cancer by **willpower"**.* This statement coming from the *personal* experience of a scientist considered the father of modern medicine, author of 33 books and more than 1,600 articles, carries an extraordinary weight.

The **Will** may be ignorant of the body processes but it is always responsible for them. The **Will** sets the state of the biosystem castle of energies whose lower energetic level, PA-CO, induces DNAs' behavior and DNAs induce that of the cellular body. In a way we may envision the **Will** as the regulator of the *abstract*, and DNAs as the regulators of the *concrete,* the physiological body. *Both linked by the castle of control energies.* The key condition for health is *to habitually maintain the correct* **Will**-*state.* Recognizing wrong **Will-states** and replacing them with healthy ones and healthy mental programs would eliminate the conditioned *abstract* abnormalities, that is, the bad habits of the **Will**. Preparation to reach the correct **Will-state** with respect to some ailment, and to *habitually maintain it,* may take training time but the actual genetic corrections shall occur in no time given the energy's speed.

Knowledge of human survival has been achieved naturally and culturally. Man avoids poisons instinctively or informed by experience. But today his own DNAs are fatally threatening his life and escape is not feasible. The author declines to bring the reader the dreadful statistics of genetic diseases *embodied* in unruled DNAs.

The next unavoidable step of medical research is the *voluntary* control of DNAs without which human survival is in danger.

VOLUNTARY CONTROL OF DNAs.

Man can learn the proper use of his **Will** to control his DNAs and *genetic* health, when provided with adequate feedback information.

The **Will,** as a top executive of a large corporation, depends on feedback information to make its decisions. It does not need to understand the technical procedures and details of its management. He relies on the results. The structure of the corporation gives the executive the *power* to control it. As in Nature's action, he is guided not by *what it is* but by *what it works*. Likewise, the **Will** has the power to make the genetic machinery work without knowing *how it works*. And for what may matter *not knowing* either how its decisions are communicated to DNAs. It is guided by feedback information that by giving the result of its decisions secures the success of them.

By far the most extraordinary factor of these processes is that the workings of **control-energies** take so diminutive amounts of physical energies. The marvels of the brain are performed with less than 25 watts. Differences of energy levels in the body's states that trigger living phenomena are not very considerable. A small variation of those levels can produce monumental changes. Genetic power is *informational* rather than *physical*! The cancer cure is not a matter of harsh or radical measures. It is a matter of precision and direction. That is, *of knowing*!

To re-establish control of abnormal DNA is *energetically* an insignificant job. Let's place it in the right perspective.

- A few rebellious DNAs are fighting against *sixty trillion* DNAs *inducing health!*

- Cancerous DNA follows *exclusively* its code of life; healthy DNAs are using theirs and mutual *collaboration*, plus the tremendous survival induction of the whole body.

- Cancerous DNA improvises a confusing local behavior in a territory that is *opposing,* by large, such changes.

- The *healthy* DNA's code is the correct one, the host, the one conditioned by timeless harmonies. Cancerous DNA's code is the *new error* unfit to the system to which is subordinated.

No wonder that cancer cells are *more vulnerable* than healthy ones to drastic treatments. They cannot subsist without the help of a <u>cancerous **Will**</u>. A cancerous **Will** is the mighty power that is on their side. It is the cancerous **Will** that in sending suicidal programs to the DNA is causing DNA to reach the point of individual rebellion. Rebel DNA now follows its own *codes of life;* the only ones left that guarantee its survival within a suicidal body. DNA does not have the proper blue print of the cellular social pattern to correct its unsocial behavior. **PA-CO has it,** but has succumbed to the overpowering inductions from above initiated by the **Will.** Abstract processes are practically *instantaneous* and DNA responds to them thanks to the extraordinary speed of its reactions.

Our present technology has the capabilities to develop instruments to reflect almost simultaneously these DNAs' responses in linear graphs or *real-time* screen images. Such instrumentation would make possible the *voluntary regulation of DNAs* by **Clinical Biofeedback.**

"Faith in healing is 50% of the cure".

A sentence similar to this one is contained in most medical books. **Clinical Genetic Feedback Instrumentation** will raise this faith to *factual evidence* by making visible the **voluntary** control of DNAs in relation to specific diseases.

INSTRUMENTATION FOR GENETIC BIOFEEDBACK.

There have been discussed in this thesis the *external orders induced* by PA-CO due to the *superiority* of genetic patterns over concrete realities. The genetic control to halt cancerous division rests in the development of **instrumentation** that will signal the relation **Will -DNAs** on the *PA-CO induced external orders*. The sharp change of cancerous DNA to a healthy one is a response to the global cancerous PA-CO matrix *reprogramming.* **Clinical Genetic Biofeedback** is based on the changes of those PA-CO patterns.

Because these *patterns* are indivisible there is no need to read the entire pattern of *induced external orders* but simply a signature of them. Once the orders, *genetically induced,* have been identified it will suffice to tap a *variable* of those orders that will show the sharp energetic change between cancerous and normal **states.** As for example: intensity, luminosity, etc., with these signals the patient will be able to adjust his **Will** to correct cancerous DNAs. Soon he will produce healthy PA-CO patterns and in time he will become conditioned **permanently** to healthy **states.** The patient will master the *voluntary* control of DNAs activities by seeing in the instrument his *capability* to control or rather induce them.

Clinical Biofeedback and Clinical Genetic Biofeedback differ only in the type of instrumentation and feedback information provided to the patient. The first gear to tap **physiological** information, the second to tap **genetic** information. Physiological control implies *genetic control.*

The genetic control by the **Will** is permanent and inescapable.

But the *direct, instantaneous genetic information for direct, instantaneous genetic control,* -**that is needed to cure cancer, AIDS and typically genetic diseases**- *that* is not detectable by any present instrument. And without it the **Will** cannot reprogram DNAs. What is the use of deciphering DNA's code if man does not know how to manipulate it? A ship without rudder! Not knowing the *genetic* consequences of his **Will** 's decisions, man does not master his body unless he will achieve the *voluntary* control of his DNAs by Clinical Genetic Biofeedback. The present *genetic* blind route has proven to be so dangerous that nobody could cross it. Cancer, AIDS and genetic diseases mean death.

The instrumentation here proposed is for general use. *The adaptation of the instrument to a specific treatment depends solely on its calibration* that should be done with healthy persons and patients with the *genetic* ailment in consideration: cancer, AIDS, schizophrenia, diabetes, etc., As a feedback signal, music being a universal language, opposed to unbearable noises, may extend the application of clinical feedback therapies to infants, mentally retarded, blind, patients and even to animals. Patients will tend invariably to seek pleasurable information avoiding an unpleasant one.

If we pause here for a second, we cannot but see that pleasure and harmony, and possibly music, is the overall fabric and drive of universal action. Negative feelings and emotions, of which fear is the most disruptive, can be interpreted as *abstract* reflections of disharmony with the Universe. Thus, the pain and discomfort from these emotional deviations are clear incitements towards correction.

Let's go back to our work.

Physiological disorders, ought to have a *genetic component* and the *same genetic biofeedback instrumentation* shall pinpoint it. In choosing the healthy group of people to establish their *inducing patterns* it is of importance to consider that a *physiological* disorder may take hours or days to appear following the *genetic* disorder. Medical history of the healthy-group must dispel the possibility to have a latent *genetic* component of the disorder that would make them useless as guidance. The good news about this *genetic-physiological* delay is that diseases can be caught at the *genetic* level before materializing into the cellular or physiological level. Therefore, Clinical Genetic Biofeedback, opening the door to the genetic ball, should prevent *physiological* disorders by timely *genetic* correction.

AIDS, A LESSER PROBLEM THAN CANCER.

The cure of AIDS should not be such a big deal as the cure of cancer considering that the AIDS virus (if such is the cause of AIDS):

- is not the formidable adversary that a cancerous DNA is with its colossal information, power and speed of reaction,

- is a foreign system to the body easier to be recognized as a threat to survival than erroneous DNA is,

- aims to the destruction of the cell instead of its prolific replication; in fact, it cannot live without stealing cell's resources that might provoke a cell's self-defense reaction at any given moment,

- is invited to lodge by a weakened *physiological* immune system rather than by a *genetic* cancerous error of superior input than any physiological action,

- genetic errors shall be reprogrammed or erased directly by **Will**, while even external agents can bust physiological immunity.

Viruses are known to be expelled by antibodies or to vanish by a strong *physiological* immune reaction triggered by vaccination. To repel AIDS requires an alert functioning of the immune system, while no such perspective appears in the horizon of cancer. Cancer is pure *genetic* error.

If cancer can be cured, surely AIDS will also!

GENETIC MEDICINE.

Upon confirmation of these ideas and techniques, necessarily, the field of Medicine will switch from the *local* and *wired-in* processes to the *patterned energies,* from the *external* remedies to the safest, fastest and most effective self-controlling techniques of *biofeedback*, from *empirical* data to *rationalized principles.*

Genetic Medicine defined, as "the **voluntary** manipulation of the **genetic** machinery to promote health" **is** the self-restructuration of a defective genetic system via the **conscious Will** and abstract resources. Hence it is *unadulterated* Medicine or self-healing. It will eliminate damages inflicted by intrusive techniques of surgery or radiation and side effects of chemotherapies, analgesics or antibiotics.

Genetic Medicine will assimilate and will eventually replace other healing disciplines, because every disorder or disease, by commission or omission, is *genetically* sustained and/or has a *genetic* origin. The significance of this approach has been implicitly gaining prominence with the fields of Psychosomatic Medicine, Psychology, Psychiatry, Noesiology, and recent Clinical Biofeedback, in the sense that these fields make *the abstract* a crucial part in the formula of healing.

Genetic Medicine, in addition, has a premonitory quality on account of the *time-interval* between *genetic* and *physiological* events, and might well be the scientific stand of preventive Medicine. On the other hand, when the body learns it never forgets, and helping to unveil its own *genetic* resources in the treatment of one specific disease could be the everlasting cure of it.

The prospect is extremely exciting for the *genetic* cures, in addition, shall be almost *instantaneous.* Once the **Will-state** of genetic correction is set, the total selection of keys to be played by every elementary function of the system is also set. Then, physical action moves faster than light, almost automatically or with a very limited margin of individual choices. Computers have familiarized us with such speeds. Should I decide to erase a word in this book, the entire transcript would edit itself to fit the alteration in **a fraction of second.** And so, my DNAs under my **Will**'s decisions.

AUTHOR'S PLEAD FOR GOVERNMENT AND PRIVATE FUNDING.

Will's decisions, thoughts and emotions are sensed and stored as memories in the DNAs becoming part of the DNAs codes that, for good or for bad, control the cells. They are a *powerful genetic reality* imposed over 60 trillion cells of the body. Poison or Life!

The cancer patient has the unprecedented mission of winning the **conscious** control of the DNAs and freeing man from the chains of genetic disorder. In his fight for survival not only will he achieve the cure of genetic diseases but also he will expand the mind and freedom of man forever.

No effort or cost should be spared in the development of Clinical Genetic Feedback **instrumentation** indispensable to conquer the *voluntary control of the genetic system*. This book is an urgent plead to government and private philanthropy for funding such an enterprise that may decide the future between two opposite ends: evolution or destruction!

ABOUT THE AUTHOR

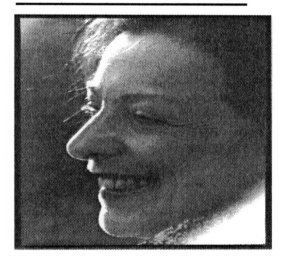

Maria L. Costell Gaydos, Doctor in Industrial
Chemistry, worked as professor assistant in the
Universities of Valencia and Barcelona (Spain) and as
Chief Chemist at Beecham Co. in Milan (Italy). In 1963
she came to USA, became American Citizen and continued
working for the chemical and pharmaceutical industries
holding positions of Senior Research Chemist at Colgate
Palmolive Research Center, Chief Chemist at Houbigant

Inc., and Director of Research at Veri-Tone Research Packaging Corp. She has been consultant and marketing researcher for several other companies and founder of Marie Louise Corp., and Cancer Studies Through Energy States Corp. She married twice having three children from her first marriage: Sergio, Giselle and David, and two from her second marriage: Paloma and Sabrina.

(Footnotes)

[1] * This departure is taken for it simplifies the task to elucidate cellular functioning by dividing it into two sections. First the study of the DNA activity and second the cell activity subordinated to the DNA control.

This thesis is ONLY concerned with the subordination of the cell to DNA. The theory of systems retains that the normal or abnormal cellular behavior results from the normal of abnormal behavior of the DNA.

The *wired-in* relation between the DNA and the cell (that is retained to be erroneous by this treatise) does not enter the picture of this book.

[2] New Mind, New Body by Barbara B. Brown, Ph.D.-Bantam Books. Edition December 1975.

[3] Am. J. Phys. Med. 1967, 46: 480-489 and 1427-1440; Science 1972, 176 : 603-609.

[4] Centro de Noesiology Dr. Escudero. Rocafort.- Valencia.- Spain. http://dr.escudero.com.

[5] Dr. Escudero's findings, based on one hundred patients operated on without anesthesia for varicose veins, were presented in the Fourth World Congress on Pain, Seattle, Washington, 1984. Another paper of about 545 varicose vein operations without anesthesia was submitted to the European Chapter of the International Society of Phlebology, London. September 1985.

Printed in the United States
21734LVS00003B/75